the
keto
diet
cookbook

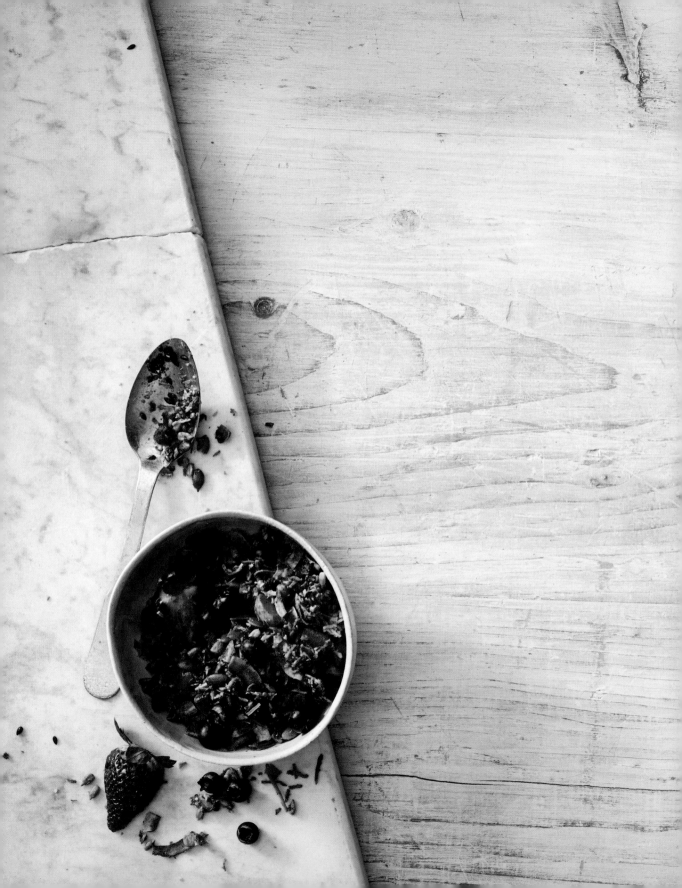

the keto diet cookbook

FROM THE BESTSELLING AUTHOR OF THE CLEAN LIVING SERIES

SCOTT GOODING

hachette
AUSTRALIA

hachette
AUSTRALIA

Published in Australia and New Zealand in 2019
by Hachette Australia
(an imprint of Hachette Australia Pty Limited)
Level 17, 207 Kent Street, Sydney NSW 2000
www.hachette.com.au

10 9 8 7 6 5 4 3 2 1

A catalogue record for this book is available from the National Library of Australia

ISBN 978 0 7336 4096 4

Cover design by Liz Seymour, Seymour Design
Internal design and layout by Liz Seymour, Seymour Design
Photography by Guy Bailey
Food styling by Jenn Tolhurst
Colour reproduction by Splitting Image
Printed in China by Toppan Leefung Printing Limited

contents

introduction

With my recent book *The Keto Diet*, my aim was to unpack the mechanics behind a low-carb diet. The book explained the benefits of embracing a low-carb or keto diet, and trust me, ketosis fuels a truckload of life-enhancing processes. Throughout, I maintained that the key to following and adhering to a healthy lifestyle hinges on building a solid foundation. The foundation of a healthy lifestyle is an acceptance of natural foods and cooking, and both of these have been neglected increasingly over the past 80 years.

OPTIMAL HEALTH

I talk a great deal about striving for optimal health, which includes cellular health and cognitive function. I'm of the contingent that believes nutrition can occupy 80 per cent of the bandwidth of optimal health, with the remaining 20 per cent comprising a number of factors. These factors can all contribute to overall health and wellbeing due to the influence they can have (collectively or in isolation) on inflammation. They include work, exercise, sleep, stress, hydration, family and friends, and can all potentially spike your stress hormones, inducing inflammation. There are a number of factors within the 20 per cent bandwidth, however, that are hard to control – for example, a stressful work email or your kids causing havoc in aisle five of the supermarket. These are external factors. If you have full control over your nutrition, the great news is that this occupies 80 per cent of the bandwidth of optimal health. You can control what passes through your lips – every nibble, bite, sip and slurp. This is an internal factor.

BEING A CUSTODIAN OF YOUR HEALTH

At no time in our history has food been more convenient. Dinner can be delivered to our front door; our weekly meals can be dropped off by any number of companies with just a few clicks of the mouse. This is all well and good (and exceptionally handy on occasion), but every time we outsource our food we relinquish control and ownership of our health. Takeaway restaurants or ready-meals companies (with the exception of a select few) don't give two hoots about our health; they are invested in producing tasty food (hopefully) and making money – nothing wrong with that, but just know that they don't have your cells' best interests at heart. To ensure the best for your cells, it's essential to be the custodian of your health, which means two things: embracing natural food and cooking at home.

WORKING YOUR KITCHEN MUSCLE

To take control and ownership of your health, the first step is to jump into the kitchen and cook up some delicious and nourishing meals. It seems pretty straightforward, but many of us in the Western world simply aren't doing this. In my experience, there are a number of reasons why people have little interest in cooking at home. I've heard many explanations over the years, but a common one is the claim that healthy food is tasteless and bland. Perhaps this was the case back in the 1970s, when the definition of healthy food was mung beans and alfalfa sprouts, but times have changed, as have science and what is now considered healthy food. To me, there's absolutely no reason for your home-cooked food to be tasteless.

Another common reason is that many of us have labelled ourselves as 'bad cooks' and simply don't cook because of it. This I can relate to, but the same rules apply to improving any skill or discipline and re-attaching a new and refreshed label. Being a good cook is very achievable; it just requires a little perseverance and an understanding of the importance of not trying to run before you can walk.

Just like if I wanted bigger biceps (and I do!) I'd go to the gym and work that particular muscle group repeatedly until it got bigger and stronger; if you want to improve your cooking skills, you need to get into the kitchen and get your hands dirty ... repeatedly. If you've labelled yourself a bad cook, messy cook or are simply not inspired to cook for yourself, then start with some basics and practise them. There's no sense in being too 'chefy', just as I wouldn't attempt to lift dumbbells that were too heavy ... I'd be smart about it and take a step-by-step approach.

AMPLIFY THE FLAVOUR OF YOUR FOOD

The key to getting you excited about your creations and inspired to cook more and more in your own kitchen is to ensure your food tastes delicious. There are plenty of tricks, hacks and strategies to boost the flavour of your home-cooking, and you certainly don't need to be a chef to adopt any of them. These tricks will transform your creation from a good dish to a great dish.

Luckily, I've done some of the hard work for you with the 150 recipes in this book – all you need to do is follow my lead. I want you to cook my recipes and enjoy them with your loved ones but, more importantly, I hope this book will be a tool from which you learn. My recipes all adhere to a particular protocol, which I outlined in *The Keto Diet*. They endorse and celebrate natural foods, good-quality protein, healthy fats, herbs and spices, and prioritise flavour and ease. I'd love for you to use these recipes as a framework from which you can create beautiful dishes independently.

KETO SNAPSHOT

If you've had the opportunity to read *The Keto Diet*, you'll have a good understanding of the mechanics of a low-carb or keto diet and how to frame your recipes, but for those of you who haven't, here's a quick overview. Essentially, the foods I'm showcasing and cooking with use ingredients that promote health and longevity as well as cognitive function. For me, the path to optimal health is related to minimising, reducing and avoiding inflammation as best you can. Some is inevitable and out of your control (that stressful work email), but a large chunk of inflammation can be controlled by you. By becoming the custodian of your own health, you will now be in the driver's seat, enabling you to navigate the current food landscape and minimise inflammatory foods.

Let's have a quick look at some of the foods that I love to cook with and which you'll find throughout the recipes. First, I'm a huge proponent of veggies – there's not one diet on this planet that advocates eating fewer veggies, and this cookbook is no different. In fact, I believe veggies should be the hero of your plate, with your protein being the 'condiment' – not the other way around. So you'll discover plenty of veggie-based recipes and in particular 'above-ground' veg. These plants are rich in the important nutrients (vitamins, minerals) which feed our biochemistry to ensure we function optimally.

I cook with and flavour food with fat from grass-fed and ethical sources. Nearly every recipe calls for a fat of some kind, whether it's butter, ghee, lard, tallow, coconut oil, avocado oil, olive oil, walnut oil or MCT oil, to name a few! My recipes are free of inflammatory fats such as industrialised seed oils for good reasons; instead, I embrace the nourishing fats mentioned above. Fat gives the dish a particular nuance as well as nutritional value, and selecting different fats to cook with will create versatility with a dish. With that in mind, feel free to be creative in the kitchen by trying various fats, simply using my recipes as a guide.

All my protein comes from ethical sources and I choose organic, grass-fed, biodynamic protein wherever possible. I always use free-range, organic eggs and Marine Stewardship Council (MSC) seafood, which is the global gold standard for sustainable seafood. It's not a prerequisite for my recipes that you shop and cook with ethical protein, as I understand that availability and cost comes into the equation. However, if we all endeavour to eat ethically whenever we can, it makes a difference to not only animal welfare and conservation, but to your cellular health.

There a few offal recipes to choose from. If you are new to offal, don't feel like you have to cook up lashings of it; instead, try including some in your regular dishes such as bolognese. It adds richness to the dish while upregulating its nutrient density.

Lastly, I'm all about simplicity and ease with cooking, but at the same time getting the maximum flavour. As I mentioned earlier, the key to getting excited about home-cooked food is to make it delicious. It needs to be alluring, sexy, inviting and comforting, so all my recipes use various ingredients to heighten the flavour, even if it's something very simple like a squeeze of lemon, a knob of butter or a herbaceous dressing. I see no point in creating healthy recipes that lack depth and flavour. We eat several times a day for our entire life, so why not make every experience a great experience? Everything that passes through our lips is not only an opportunity to enhance and amplify our health but also a chance to excite our tastebuds.

THE KETO DIET COOKBOOK FORTNIGHT EATING PLAN

I've included a two-week eating plan simply to provide you with a framework to work from. Just as I did in *The Keto Diet*, I've composed this meal plan as scaffolding for you to build your own eating plan. By no means is anything set in stone, so feel free to customise your fortnight. The wonderful thing with this type of eating plan is that you have the freedom to chop and change as you please. The ingredients and macronutrients I've focused on are designed to nourish and enhance your health and not be a metabolic burden. A diet rich in carbohydrates and/or refined foods carries with it a hormonal or metabolic cost. It's worth noting at this point that following a lifestyle as depicted in this cookbook or in *The Keto Diet* can also help to normalise hormone regulation. It is our hormones that are responsible for the partitioning of energy, and ultimately ill-health and weight gain if normal regulation is disrupted.

I hope you enjoy the recipes in this book and that they encourage you to experiment with nourishing and flavourful foods. You never know, you might just strike GOLD!

Happy cooking – Scott x

the
fortnight
eating
plan

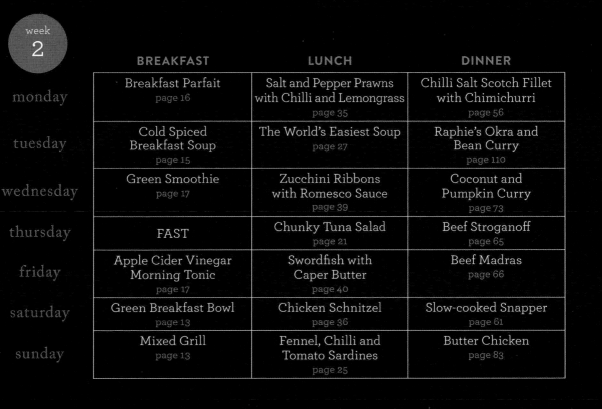

week 1

	BREAKFAST	LUNCH	DINNER
monday	Duck Egg Omelette page 10	Chicken Tacos page 29	Pork Chops with Celeriac and Carrot Mash page 110
tuesday	Scrambled Eggs with Kale and Onion Pesto page 9	Barbecued Banana Prawns with Herb Mayo page 39	Rump Steak with Anchovy Butter page 56
wednesday	FAST	Green Mango Salad page 21	Goat Curry page 47
thursday	Pink Smoothie page 18	Flaked Salmon with Mediterranean Medley page 43	Lamb Chops with Garlic and Mint dressing page 90
friday	Bulletproof Coffee with Cinnamon page 18	Crispy Grilled Sardines with Parsley Dressing page 25	Whole Baked Snapper with Nuoc Cham page 85
saturday	Granola with Berries page 9	Prawn and Egg Tacos page 44	Moules Mariniere page 48
sunday	Cacao Smoothie page 17	20-minute Chicken page 40	Beef Rogan Josh page 51

week 2

	BREAKFAST	LUNCH	DINNER
monday	Breakfast Parfait page 16	Salt and Pepper Prawns with Chilli and Lemongrass page 35	Chilli Salt Scotch Fillet with Chimichurri page 56
tuesday	Cold Spiced Breakfast Soup page 15	The World's Easiest Soup page 27	Raphie's Okra and Bean Curry page 110
wednesday	Green Smoothie page 17	Zucchini Ribbons with Romesco Sauce page 39	Coconut and Pumpkin Curry page 73
thursday	FAST	Chunky Tuna Salad page 21	Beef Stroganoff page 65
friday	Apple Cider Vinegar Morning Tonic page 17	Swordfish with Caper Butter page 40	Beef Madras page 66
saturday	Green Breakfast Bowl page 13	Chicken Schnitzel page 36	Slow-cooked Snapper page 61
sunday	Mixed Grill page 13	Fennel, Chilli and Tomato Sardines page 25	Butter Chicken page 83

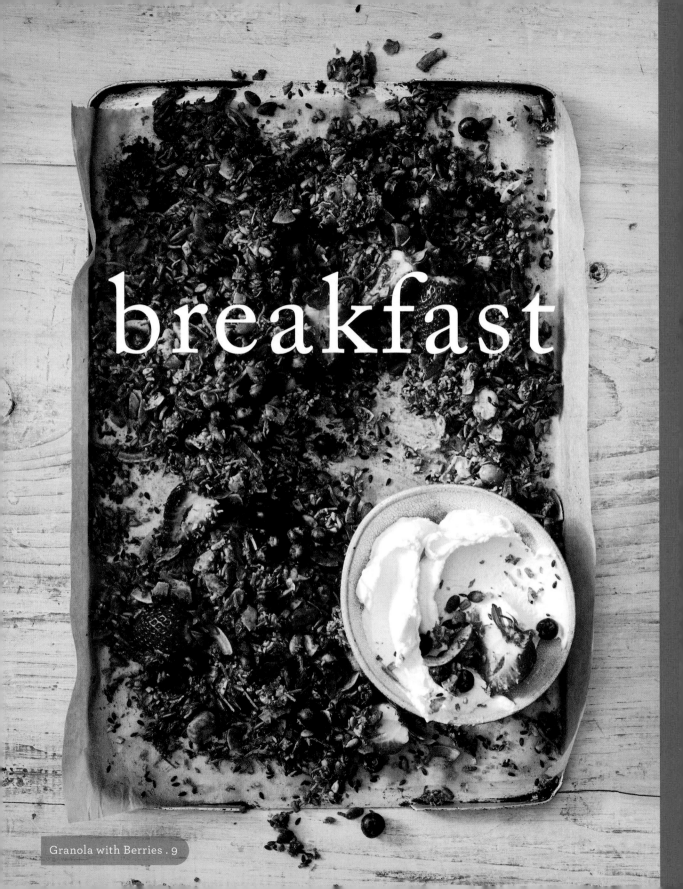

breakfast

serves
4

Granola with Berries

If you're craving crunch at the breakfast table, this granola will tick that box, plus you can throw it in to Scott Gooding's Mess (see recipe page 151) or any smoothie for some added texture.

2 cups coconut flakes
½ cup pepitas
½ cup sunflower seeds
½ cup walnuts
½ cup pecans
2 tablespoons linseeds
½ cup macadamias
1 teaspoon cinnamon
1 teaspoon allspice
2–3 tablespoons coconut oil
1 tablespoon honey
1 cup coconut yoghurt, to serve
1 cup fresh or frozen berries, to serve

1   Preheat your oven to 180°C and line two baking trays with baking paper.

2   In a large mixing bowl, combine all the dry ingredients including the spices. Add the coconut oil and honey and combine thoroughly.

3   Spread the granola evenly onto the baking trays and bake for 15 minutes, swapping trays at midway point.

4   Remove from the oven and allow to cool. Serve with coconut yoghurt and berries.

serves
2

Scrambled Eggs with Kale and Onion Pesto

I love this recipe – it's a fabulous departure from ordinary scrambled eggs. Slow-cooking the kale and onions adds a beautiful sweetness to the eggs.

2 tablespoons ghee (or more if needed)
1 brown onion, chopped
4–5 kale leaves, trimmed and chopped
6 eggs
sea salt and freshly ground black pepper, to taste

1   Place a frying pan over low heat and add 1 tablespoon of the ghee. Add the onion and sauté for 4–5 minutes, stirring occasionally. Add the kale and cook for a further 4–5 minutes, or until softened, adding more ghee if needed.

2   Remove from the pan and place in a blender. Blitz for 30 seconds, or until fully combined.

3   Place your frying pan back over low heat and add the remaining ghee. In a bowl, gently whisk the eggs and add to the pan. Add 2–3 tablespoons of the onion pesto to the eggs and stir using a wooden spoon. Cook for 3–4 minutes, or until eggs are cooked to your liking.

4   Remove from the heat, season with salt and pepper, and serve.

serves
2

Duck Egg Omelette

Don't sweat it if you can't get hold of duck eggs, just use your usual organic chicken eggs, but add another egg.

1 tablespoon duck fat or ghee
½ brown onion, chopped
handful of mushrooms, roughly chopped
1 teaspoon chilli flakes
handful of rocket
3 duck or 4 chicken eggs
sea salt and freshly ground black
   pepper, to taste

1   Place a large frying pan over medium heat and add the fat or ghee. Add the onion and cook for 1 minute.

2   Add the mushrooms and chilli and cook for 3–4 minutes. As they begin to soften, add the rocket and stir through.

3   Gently whisk the duck eggs in a bowl and add to the frying pan, then reduce the heat to low. Cook until the omelette is browned on the underside, then flip it over and cook to your liking. Season with salt and pepper, and serve.

serves
4

Keto Kedgeree

Traditionally, kedgeree is made with rice, spices and smoked fish. This is a low-carb version and tastes great. It works well any time of the day, too, not just at breakfast!

350 g cauliflower, stalks and leaves
   trimmed
2 tablespoons butter
2 garlic cloves, chopped
1 brown onion, chopped
3 shallots, trimmed and chopped
1 teaspoon cumin
1 teaspoon curry powder
1 teaspoon turmeric
400 g smoked fish (remove any skin or bones)
150 g English spinach, roughly chopped
sea salt and freshly ground black pepper,
   to taste
2 soft-boiled eggs, halved

1   Blitz the cauliflower in a food processor to form rice. Remove from the jug and set aside.

2   Place a large frying pan over low heat and add the butter. Add the garlic, onion and shallots and sauté for 4–6 minutes, or until softened. Add the cumin, curry powder and turmeric, and stir for 1 minute.

3   Add the cauliflower rice and cook, stirring, for 2–3 minutes.

4   Add the smoked fish and cook for 4–5 minutes.

5   Add the spinach and cook until wilted and the cauliflower is warmed through.

6   Remove from the heat, season with salt and pepper, and serve with the boiled eggs.

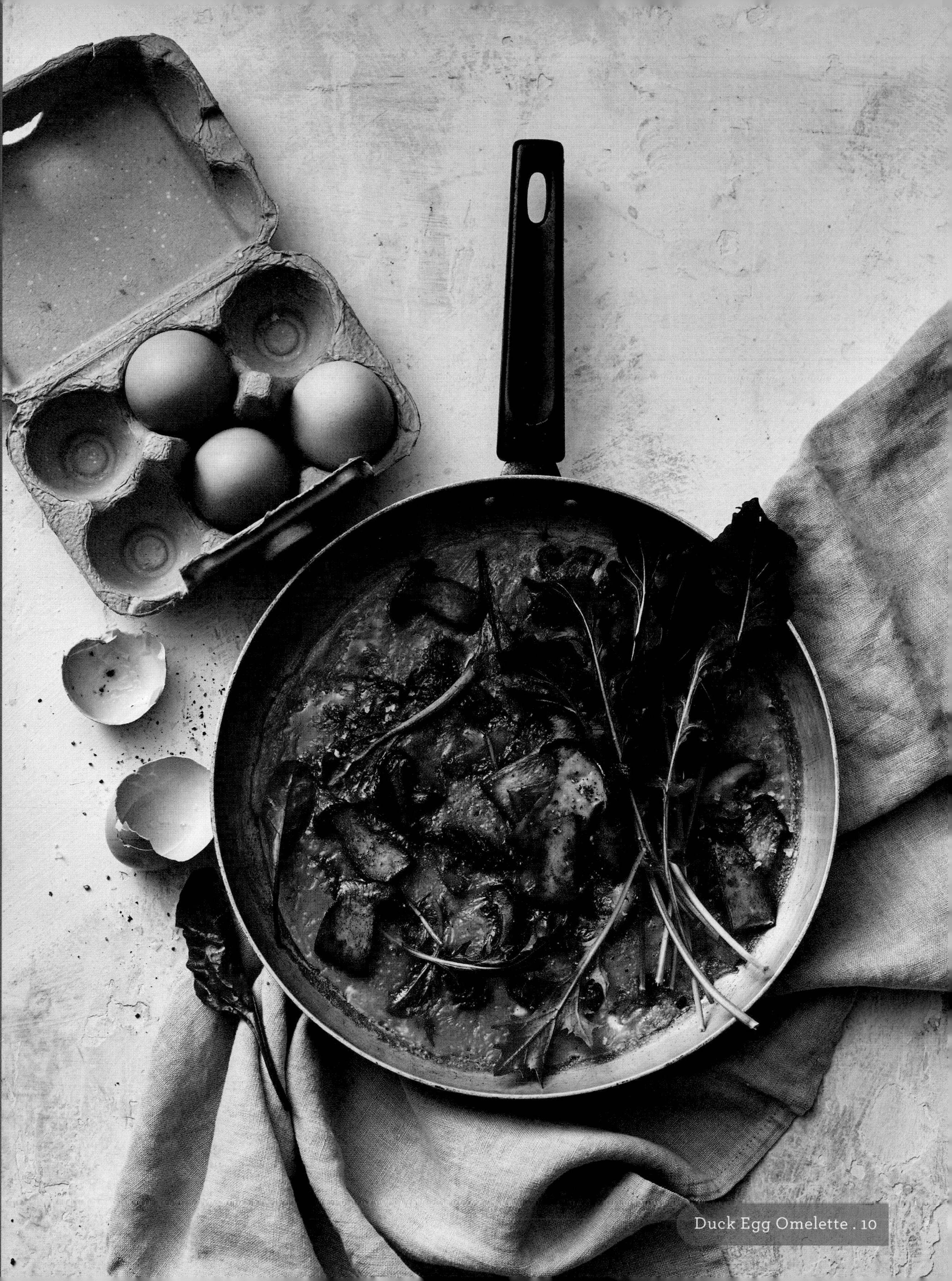

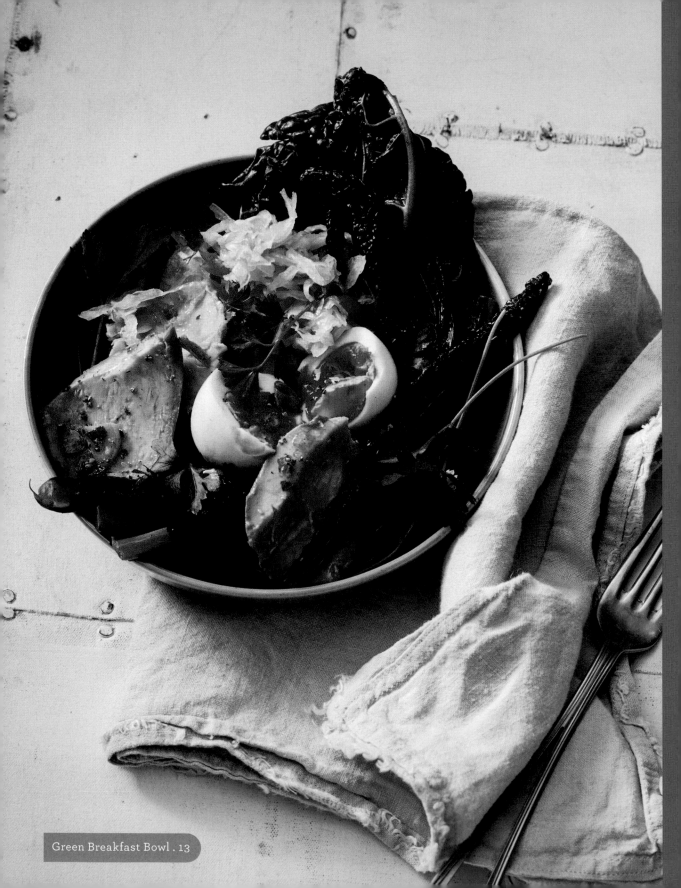

Green Breakfast Bowl . 13

serves
2

serves
1

Green Breakfast Bowl

This is a great recipe that doesn't have to be for breakfast – you can whip it up any time of the day. Sauerkraut is a healthy addition to any salad.

2 tablespoons coconut oil
⅓ bunch of Tuscan kale, trimmed
   and roughly chopped
2 garlic cloves, sliced
½ teaspoon chilli flakes
2 eggs
½ avocado, cut in wedges
2 tablespoons Sauerkraut
   (see recipe page 118)
handful of snow pea sprouts
juice of 1 lemon
1 tablespoon olive oil
sea salt and freshly ground black
   pepper, to taste

1   Place a frying pan over medium heat and add the coconut oil. Add the kale, garlic and chilli and sauté for 4–5 minutes, or until softened. Remove from the heat and set aside.

2   Place the eggs in a small saucepan, cover with cold water and bring to the boil. Reduce the heat to a simmer and cook for 6 minutes (soft boiled). Remove the eggs, run under cold water and peel.

3   In a large bowl, combine the kale mixture with the avocado wedges, sauerkraut, snow pea sprouts and eggs.

4   Drizzle with lemon juice and olive oil, season with salt and pepper, and serve.

Mixed Grill

I'm revealing my English roots with this recipe, but this hearty English breakfast is back on the popular list. The 'greasy fry-up', as it used to be called, can be healthy if it's cooked with healthful fats such as coconut oil or butter.

2 teaspoons olive oil
handful of cherry tomatoes
2 gluten-free sausages
2 rashers of bacon
1 egg
handful of baby spinach leaves
sea salt and freshly ground black
   pepper, to taste

1   Place a small saucepan over low heat and add 1 teaspoon of the olive oil. Add the tomatoes and cook for 3–4 minutes, stirring occasionally.

2   Place a large frying pan over high heat, add the remaining olive oil and cook the sausages until browned all over. Add the bacon to the pan and cook for 3–4 minutes on either side, or to your liking. Remove the sausages and bacon from the pan and set aside.

3   Crack the egg into the frying pan and cook to your liking. Remove from the heat.

4   Add the spinach to the tomatoes, stir and cook for 1–2 minutes. Remove from the heat.

5   Season the tomatoes and spinach with salt and pepper, and serve with the egg, sausage and bacon.

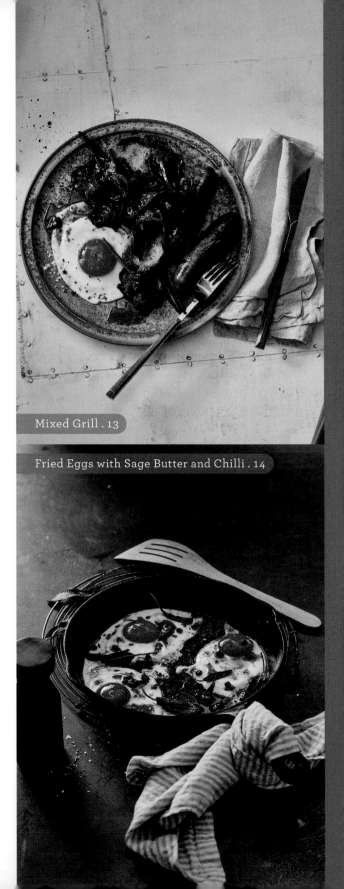

Mixed Grill . 13

Fried Eggs with Sage Butter and Chilli . 14

serves
2

Fried Eggs with
Sage Butter and Chilli

A plain ol' fried egg is delicious as it is, but
the addition of sage butter and chilli elevates
it to the next level ... enjoy!

3 tablespoons butter
4 sage leaves
4 eggs
1 long red chilli, deseeded and chopped
1 teaspoon baby capers, rinsed and
   drained
sea salt and freshly ground black
   pepper, to taste

1   Place a frying pan over low–medium
    heat and add the butter. Stir in the sage
    leaves and, once the butter begins to
    brown, remove from the pan and set
    aside somewhere warm.

2   Place your frying pan back over low–
    medium heat and add 1 tablespoon of the
    browned butter. Crack the eggs into the
    pan. Sprinkle the chilli and capers over
    the eggs. Spoon the remaining browned
    butter over the eggs while they are
    cooking. Cook until the whites are firm
    and the yolks are to your liking.

3   Remove from the heat, season with salt
    and pepper, and serve.

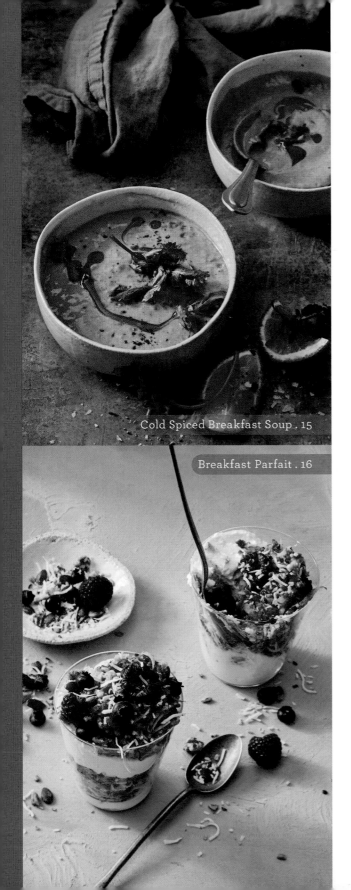

Cold Spiced Breakfast Soup . 15

Breakfast Parfait . 16

Cold Spiced Breakfast Soup

Perhaps not your immediate thought when it comes to breakfast, but this soup has all the essential ingredients to keep you feeling full and satisfied.

2 ripe avocados, flesh scooped out
600 ml coconut milk
juice of ½ lemon
1 teaspoon turmeric
½ teaspoon cumin
¼ bunch of coriander, leaves only
1 tablespoon olive oil
sea salt and freshly ground black
    pepper, to taste

1   Place all the ingredients in a blender or food processor and blitz for 30 seconds or until smooth.

2   Season again with salt and pepper if needed, and serve immediately, or place in the fridge for 30 minutes to chill.

serves
2

serves
1

Breakfast Parfait

This great breakfast recipe is keto friendly, but perhaps pop it up your sleeve for special mornings due to the carbs in the apple. Plenty of fat from the coconut cream and seeds, but also some sweetness from the apple and carrots, makes this delicious.

250 ml coconut cream
1 green apple, shredded
2 small carrots, grated
½ cup walnuts, crushed
¼ cup pepitas
¼ cup hemp seeds
½ cup shredded coconut
grated zest of 1 lemon
¼ cup blueberries

1 Chill the coconut cream in the fridge for a minimum of 2 hours. Drain the watery component from the solid cream.

2 In a large mixing bowl, combine the apple, carrot, walnuts, pepitas, hemp seeds and shredded coconut.

3 Combine the coconut cream with the lemon zest.

4 Place alternate layers of the apple/carrot mix and coconut cream in a serving glass to create a beautiful layered stack. Top with blueberries, and serve.

Macadamia Smoothie

Macadamia is one of the royalty of nuts for its omega 3:6 ratio. If you're looking for savoury macadamia recipes, check out Macadamia Pesto (page 121) and Macadamia 'Cheese' (page 128).

250 ml coconut cream
1 tablespoon macadamia butter
¼ cup macadamias
1 tablespoon pepitas
1 tablespoon hemp seeds
1 tablespoon MCT oil
30 g protein powder
handful of ice

1 Throw all the ingredients in a blender and blitz for 20 seconds or until fully combined.

2 Pour into a glass and serve.

serves
1

Cacao Smoothie

250 ml coconut milk
1 tablespoon cashew butter
1 tablespoon MCT oil
30 g vanilla protein powder
2 tablespoons cacao powder
2 tablespoons shredded coconut
handful of ice

1   Throw all the ingredients in a blender
    and blitz for 20 seconds or until smooth.

2   Pour into a glass and serve.

serves
1

Apple Cider Vinegar
Morning Tonic

This drink won't stimulate your insulin so
won't necessarily break your morning fast,
but it will kickstart the digestive enzymes
in your gut and liver.

2 tablespoons apple cider vinegar
    (containing mother)
½ teaspoon turmeric
glass of cold water

1   Stir the vinegar and turmeric into the
    glass of water and drink.

serves
1

Green Smoothie

Even though my smoothies are high
fat and low carb, I still cram a heap of
greens into most of them.

250 ml coconut milk or cream
½ ripe avocado, flesh scooped out
1 tablespoon nut butter of your choice
1 tablespoon MCT oil
⅓ bunch of English spinach
30 g vanilla protein powder
¼ Jerusalem artichoke
1 tablespoon pepitas
handful of ice
splash of water if needed

1   Throw all the ingredients in a blender
    and blitz for 20 seconds or until fully
    combined.

2   Pour into a glass and serve.

Bulletproof Coffee with Cinnamon

This style of coffee will put hairs on your chest and certainly help you get into ketosis.

1 tablespoon butter
1 tablespoon MCT oil
1 teaspoon cinnamon
1 long black coffee

1   Throw all the ingredients in a blender and blitz for 10–15 seconds or until fully combined.

2   Pour into a glass or mug and serve.

Pink Smoothie

This is a doozy of a smoothie, with plenty of nutrients and a little sweetness from the beetroot.

250 ml coconut milk or cream
1 tablespoon nut butter of your choice
1 tablespoon MCT oil
1 tablespoon hemp oil
1 baby beetroot, trimmed
1 tablespoon shredded coconut
2 tablespoons walnuts
1 cup baby spinach leaves
30 g vanilla protein powder
handful of ice
splash of water if needed

1   Throw all the ingredients in a blender and blitz for 20 seconds or until fully combined.

2   Pour into a glass and serve.

Macadamia Smoothie . 16   Pink Smoothie . 18   Green Smoothie . 17

lunch

Simple Chunky Tuna Salad . 21

Green Mango Salad

There's something very addictive about a green mango salad; it's all in the dressing and the balance of flavours – so delicious!

2 teaspoons shrimp paste
juice of 1 lime
1 teaspoon honey
2 shallots, trimmed and chopped
1 green mango, flesh julienned
½ red onion, sliced
large handful of cherry tomatoes, halved
1 long green chilli, deseeded and finely
  chopped
1 bird's-eye chilli, finely chopped
¼ bunch of coriander, leaves picked
¼ bunch of mint, leaves picked

1   Place a frying pan over medium heat and sauté the shrimp paste for 1 minute. Remove from the heat.

2   In a small bowl, combine the shrimp paste, lime juice and honey (add more lime juice to taste if needed).

3   Place all the ingredients in a large bowl, add the dressing and gently toss to combine.

Simple Chunky Tuna Salad

This could be described as an 'unfancy' poke bowl, as it has some poke elements, but it's designed to be fuss-free and quick. If you don't have access to fresh albacore tuna, simply grab some tinned tuna instead.

500 g fresh albacore tuna, cut into chunks
  (or 500g canned tuna)
1 red onion, sliced
2 ripe avocadoes, cut into chunks
1 shallot, trimmed and chopped
1 tablespoon sesame seeds
¼ bunch of coriander, chopped
1 Lebanese cucumber, chopped

DRESSING
1 garlic clove, finely chopped
5 cm knob of ginger, finely chopped
1 small red chilli, deseeded and finely chopped
1 tablespoon lime juice
1 tablespoon fish sauce
1 teaspoon honey

1   To make the dressing, combine all the ingredients in a small jar, cover and shake vigorously. Set aside.

2   In a large mixing bowl, combine all the ingredients for the salad and lightly toss together.

3   Add the dressing and lightly toss again. Spoon into serving bowls.

serves
4

Tuna Niçoise

100 g green beans, trimmed
2 eggs
1 teaspoon olive oil
500 g albacore tuna
sea salt and freshly ground black
    pepper, to taste
1 small cos lettuce
1 punnet of medley cherry tomatoes
⅓ cup black olives, pitted
100 g anchovy fillets

DRESSING
1 teaspoon Dijon mustard
2 tablespoons apple cider vinegar
5-6 tablespoons olive oil
1 teaspoon lemon juice
handful of parsley leaves, chopped
sea salt and freshly ground black
    pepper, to taste

1   To make the dressing, place all the
    ingredients in a small jar, cover and shake
    vigorously. Set aside.

2   Bring a saucepan of salted water to the
    boil, turn off heat and add the beans. Leave
    for 4-5 minutes before draining.

3   Boil the eggs for 6 minutes then remove
    them and place in cold water. Once cooled,
    peel and halve the eggs.

4   Place a griddle pan over high heat and
    add the olive oil. Season the tuna with salt
    and pepper, and place in the pan. Cook for
    45 seconds on each side then remove from
    the heat and set aside to rest.

5   Place the salad ingredients in a large
    bowl, add the dressing and lightly toss to
    combine. Season as desired.

serves
2

Marinated Fresh Anchovy Fillets

If you choose to eat fish, then fish like
anchovy, sardines and mackerel will
certainly help you attain ketosis. They
will also contribute to your overall health.

400 g fresh anchovy fillets
150 ml white wine vinegar
3 tablespoons olive oil
grated zest of 1 lemon
1 garlic clove, finely chopped
¼ bunch of parsley, chopped
sea salt and freshly ground black
    pepper, to taste

1   In a bowl, combine the anchovy fillets
    with the vinegar, cover with plastic wrap
    and refrigerate for 4 hours.

2   Take the fillets out of the fridge and rinse
    them under cold water to remove the
    vinegar.

3   In another bowl, combine the olive oil,
    lemon zest, garlic and parsley and gently
    stir to combine.

4   Place the fillets on a large plate and drizzle
    the herb oil over them. Cover and pop in
    the fridge for 1 hour.

5   Remove the fillets from the fridge, season
    with salt and pepper, and serve.

Marinated Fresh Anchovy Fillets . 22

Crispy Grilled Sardines with Parsley Dressing . 25

serves
2

serves
2

Crispy Grilled Sardines with Parsley Dressing

Fatty fish such as sardines work so nicely with this herbaceous, acidic dressing.

12 whole sardines
1–2 tablespoons olive oil
sea salt and freshly ground black
 pepper, to taste
juice of ½ lemon

PARSLEY DRESSING
1 tablespoon lemon juice
3 tablespoons olive oil
¼ bunch of parsley, roughly chopped
sea salt and freshly ground black
 pepper, to taste

1 Place the sardines on a baking tray, drizzle with the olive oil and season with salt and pepper.

2 Preheat a grill to high and grill the sardines for 2–3 minutes on each side, or until cooked through and crispy. Remove from the heat and set aside.

3 To make the dressing, combine all the ingredients in a small glass jar, cover and shake vigorously.

4 Drizzle the lemon juice over the fish, followed by the dressing. Season with salt and pepper, and serve.

Fennel, Chilli and Tomato Sardines

Oozing with simplicity, ease and flavour, this recipe will look and taste delicious.

12 whole sardines
3 baby fennel bulbs, trimmed, cored
 and sliced
2 punnets of cherry tomatoes, halved
3 tablespoons olive oil
grated zest of 1 lemon
1 teaspoon chilli flakes
2 lemons, halved
sea salt and freshly ground black
 pepper, to taste

1 Preheat your oven to 180°C.

2 In a large baking tray, place the sardines side by side in rows, and place the fennel and tomatoes between the fish.

3 In a bowl, combine the olive oil, lemon zest and chilli flakes. Pour over the fish, fennel and tomatoes. Add the lemon halves to the tray.

4 Season with salt and pepper and bake for 10–12 minutes (times vary depending on the size of the fish).

Mushroom Soup

Here's a fun fact for you: 25 per cent
of the earth's biomass (all living things)
belong to the mushroom/fungi family.

2 tablespoons butter
1 brown onion, chopped
2 teaspoons dried thyme
1 teaspoon dried sage
500 g mixed mushrooms, chopped or left
    whole (depending on type of mushroom)
500 ml coconut cream
500 ml vegetable or chicken broth or stock
juice of ½ lemon
sea salt and freshly ground black
    pepper, to taste

1   Place a saucepan over medium heat and
    add the butter. Add the onion and sauté for
    3–4 minutes. Add the thyme and sage and
    cook for a further 1 minute.

2   Add the mushrooms and stir to coat them
    in onion, herbs and butter.

3   Add the coconut cream and the broth, and
    bring to the boil. Reduce the heat to low
    and simmer until the soup reaches your
    desired consistency.

4   Remove from the heat, add the lemon juice,
    season with salt and pepper and serve.

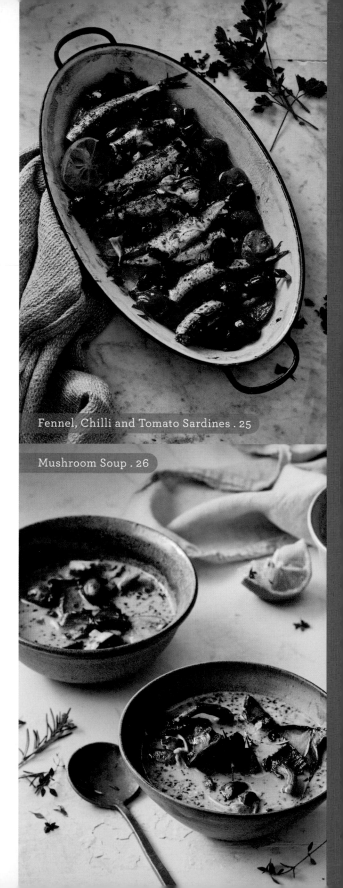

Fennel, Chilli and Tomato Sardines . 25

Mushroom Soup . 26

theketodietcookbook

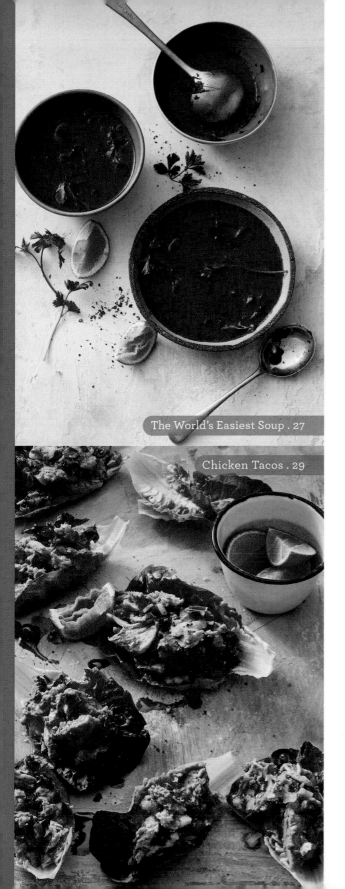

The World's Easiest Soup . 27

Chicken Tacos . 29

serves
2

The World's Easiest Soup

The backbone of any good soup, casserole or stew is a bone broth. Either invest in making your own or choose an organic, grass-fed version.

600 ml chicken or vegetable broth
  or stock
1 tablespoon ghee
3–4 leaves of silverbeet or spinach
¼ bunch of parsley
sea salt and freshly ground black
  pepper, to taste

1 Place the broth in a saucepan and bring to the boil. Remove from the heat and pour into a blender (not more than half full).

2 Add the remaining ingredients to the blender.

3 Place your hand over the lid of the blender and blitz for 20–30 seconds, or until mostly blended.

4 Return to the saucepan with the remaining broth, season with salt and pepper, stir well and serve.

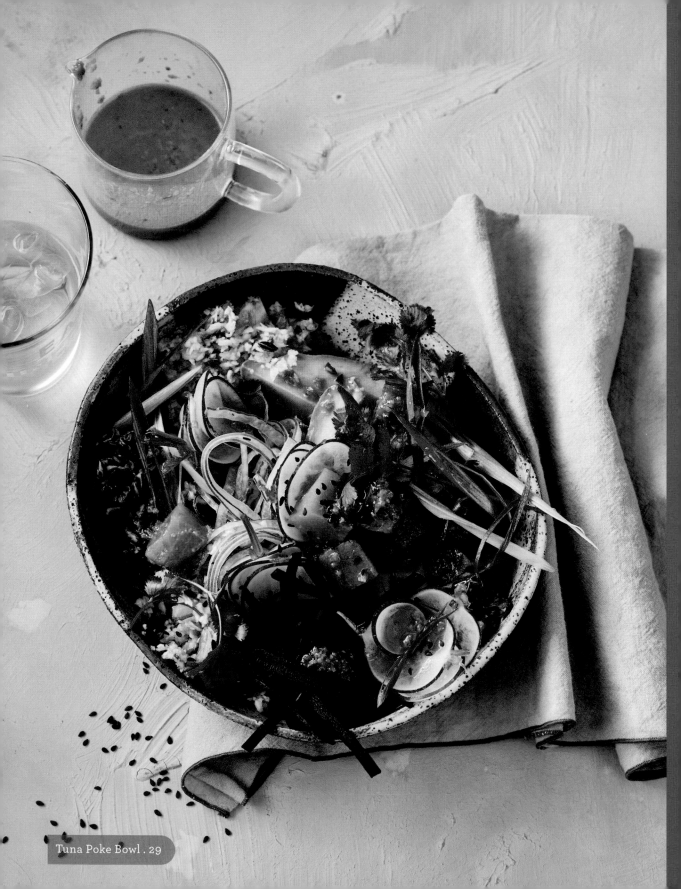

Tuna Poke Bowl . 29

Chicken Tacos

These are designed to be fun – great for getting the kids involved! Feel free to use any lettuce for this dish.

3 ripe avocados, flesh scooped out
1 small red onion, finely chopped
juice of 2 limes
2 tomatoes, seeds removed, flesh diced
500 g shredded cooked chicken
¼ bunch of coriander, leaves picked
sea salt and freshly ground black pepper,
    to taste
8 baby radicchio leaves
8 baby cos leaves

1   In a large mixing bowl, mash the avocado using a fork. Add the onion, lime juice, tomato, chicken and coriander leaves, and gently stir to combine. Season with salt and pepper.

2   Place 1–2 tablespoons of the chicken mix into each leaf cup, and serve.

Tuna Poke Bowl

In my mind there are few rules to making a poke bowl – as long as there is an array of colours, textures and flavours, you can't go wrong. What it will need, though, is a yummy dressing to bring it all together.

1 teaspoon olive oil
1 fresh albacore tuna steak
½ cup shredded green cabbage
½ cup shredded red cabbage
2 pink radishes, sliced
1 avocado, mashed
½ red onion, sliced
2 shallots, trimmed and chopped
1 small beetroot, grated

DRESSING
½ red onion, finely chopped
1 garlic clove, finely chopped
3 tablespoons olive oil
1 tablespoon lemon juice
1 tablespoon apple cider vinegar
1 tablespoon tamari
1 green chilli, finely chopped

1   To make the dressing, place all the ingredients in a mixing bowl, stir to combine and set aside.

2   Place a griddle pan over high heat and add the olive oil. Add the tuna steak and cook for 2–3 minutes on each side. Remove from the pan, allow to cool then dice.

3   In a large bowl, combine the remaining ingredients and add the diced tuna. Add 4 tablespoons of the dressing and lightly toss to combine.

serves
4

Green Bowl
with Green Tahini

What I love about this bowl is its versatility.
Feel free to substitute the greens that you have
at hand or that need using up in the fridge.

4 eggs
1 cup broccoli florets
4 kale leaves, trimmed and chopped
¼ bunch of mint, roughly chopped
¼ bunch of coriander, roughly chopped
large handful of roughly chopped endive,
    or loose salad leaves
2 tablespoons olive oil
juice of 1 lemon
sea salt and freshly ground black
    pepper, to taste
⅓ cup walnuts, lightly crushed
3 tablespoons Green Tahini
    (see recipe page 131)

1   Place the eggs in a small saucepan, cover
    with cold salted water and bring to the boil.
    Reduce the heat to a simmer and cook for
    6 minutes (soft boiled). Remove the eggs
    (keep the water simmering) and run under
    cold water. Once cooled, peel and halve
    the eggs.

2   Meanwhile, add the broccoli to the salted
    water and cook for 4–5 minutes. Drain and
    set aside to cool.

3   In a large mixing bowl, combine the kale,
    mint, coriander and endive and lightly toss
    together. Add the cooled broccoli.

4   Dress the greens with the olive oil and
    lemon juice, and season with salt and
    pepper. Sprinkle over the crushed walnuts
    and serve with the green tahini and
    boiled eggs.

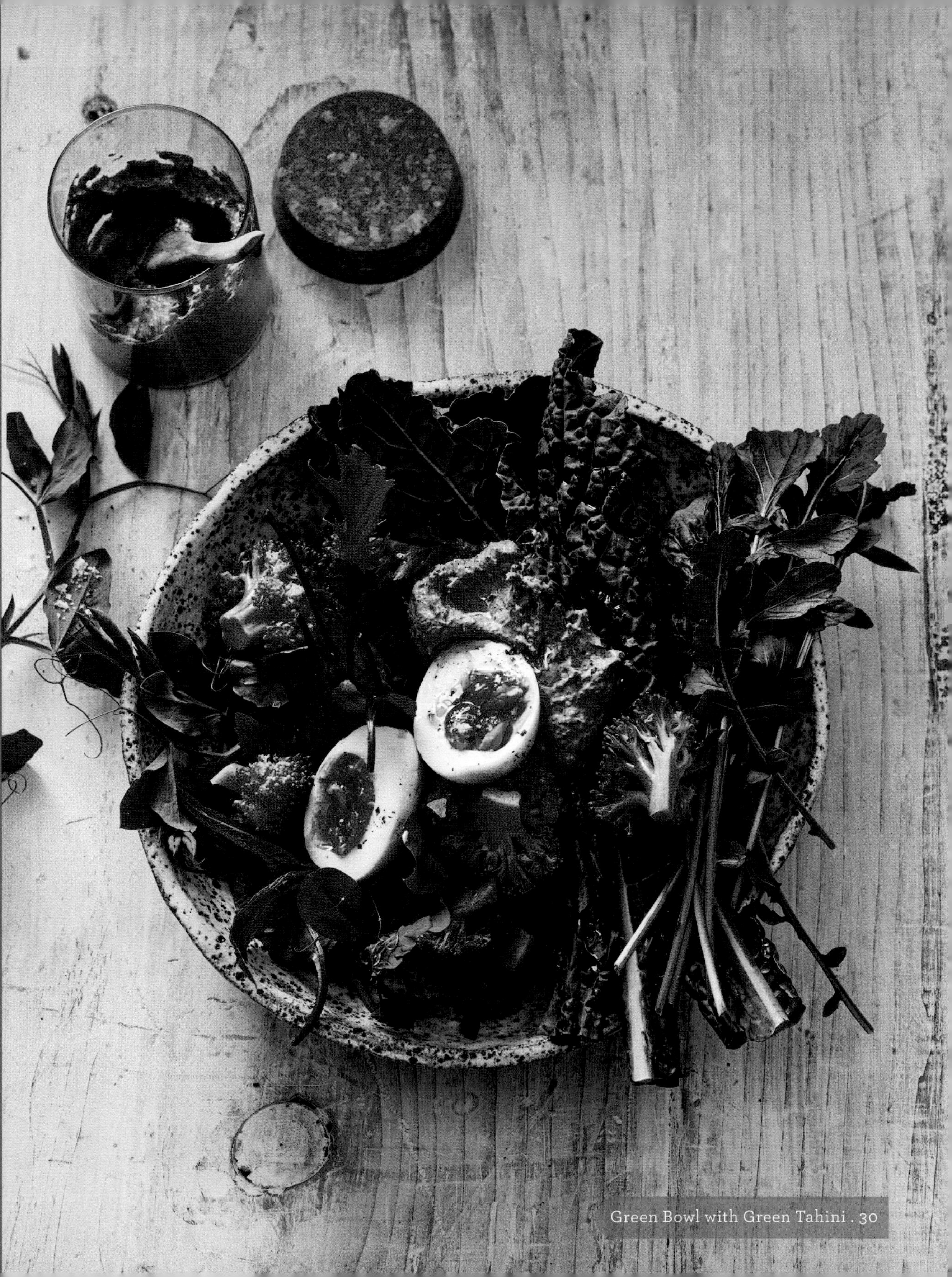

Green Bowl with Green Tahini . 30

Green Bowl with Nuoc Cham . 33

serves
2

Green Bowl
with Nuoc Cham

This light salad works well as a side,
or if you'd like it to be a more robust
and hearty meal then simply add some
sardines or tuna.

2 avocados, sliced
4 shallots, trimmed and sliced
2 little gem lettuces, leaves trimmed
¼ bunch of coriander, roughly chopped
¼ cup pepitas
6 Thai basil leaves, roughly chopped
3 tablespoons Nuoc Cham
   (see recipe page 85)
sea salt and freshly ground black
   pepper, to taste

1   In a large mixing bowl, combine all the
    ingredients for the salad and gently toss
    together.

2   Add the Nuoc Cham dressing and lightly
    toss again. Season with salt and pepper,
    and serve.

serves
4

Vegetarian Crêpes
with Satay Sauce

I'm happy eating this satay sauce by the
spoonful, so swapping a spoon for a crêpe
makes for a delicious lunch or snack.

6 eggs
sea salt and freshly ground black
   pepper, to taste
1 tablespoon coconut oil
1 carrot, julienned
1 baby fennel bulb, julienned
1 Lebanese cucumber, julienned
½ cup mint leaves
½ cup coriander leaves
¼ cup crushed cashews
1 cup Keto Satay Sauce
   (see recipe page 130)

1   Whisk the eggs with ⅓ cup of water until
    well combined. Season with salt and pepper.

2   Place a large non-stick frying pan over
    medium heat. Add some of the coconut oil
    to the pan and pour in one-quarter of the
    egg mixture to form a thin omelette. Cook
    for 1 minute then flip over. Once cooked on
    both sides, transfer the omelette to a sheet
    of baking paper. Repeat with the remaining
    egg mixture.

3   Top each omelette with carrot, fennel,
    cucumber, mint, coriander and cashews.
    Roll up to enclose the filling, and cut into
    segments.

4   Serve the rolls with warmed satay sauce.

serves
4

Pumpkin Soup
with Crispy Bacon

Warming and comforting, this recipe is
certainly one to soothe your soul.

2 tablespoons olive oil
1 large brown onion, chopped
4 garlic cloves, chopped
2 celery stalks, sliced
2 carrots, sliced
2 bay leaves
1 sprig of thyme
1 teaspoon dried sage
2 litres chicken or vegetable broth or stock
½ large pumpkin, peeled and roughly
   chopped
200–300 g short back bacon
½ bunch of parsley, roughly chopped
200 ml coconut cream (optional)
juice of ½ lemon
sea salt and freshly ground black
   pepper, to taste

1   Place a large saucepan over low–medium
    heat and add the olive oil. Add the onion,
    garlic, celery, carrots and herbs and sauté
    for 5–6 minutes.

2   Add the broth and cook for a further
    10 minutes.

3   Add the pumpkin and simmer for a further
    10–15 minutes, or until the pumpkin
    begins to soften.

4   Remove from the heat and blitz in a food
    processor or blender (you may need to do
    this in batches). Return the soup to the
    saucepan over a low heat.

5   Meanwhile, place a frying pan over
    medium–high heat and add the bacon.
    Cook for 2–3 minutes on each side, or until
    the fat has rendered and the bacon has
    gone crispy. Remove from the heat, allow
    to cool then roughly chopped the bacon.

6   Remove the soup from the heat. Add the
    parsley, bacon and coconut cream, if using,
    and stir through with the lemon juice.
    Season with salt and pepper, and serve.

Salt and Pepper Prawns with Chilli and Lemongrass

Crispy, salty and spicy is a wicked combination – the dipping sauce is the cherry on top!

⅓ cup arrowroot
1 tablespoon white pepper
1 tablespoon sea salt
1 tablespoon freshly ground black pepper
24 raw banana prawns, deveined, tails on
3 tablespoons coconut oil
1 long red chilli, sliced
1 long green chilli, sliced
2 stalks of lemongrass, white parts only, thinly sliced
4 shallots, trimmed and chopped
¼ bunch of coriander, roughly chopped
2 limes, cut into wedges

DIPPING SAUCE
1 small red chilli, finely chopped
1 garlic clove, finely chopped
1 tablespoon finely chopped ginger
1 tablespoon fish sauce
1 teaspoon honey
juice of 2 limes

1   Combine the arrowroot, white pepper, sea salt and black pepper in a large mixing bowl. Add the prawns and toss to ensure they are evenly coated.

2   Place a large frying pan over high heat and add the coconut oil. Add the chillies and lemongrass and stir-fry for 30 seconds.

3   Add the prawns and stir-fry for 2–3 minutes, or until cooked and crispy.

4   Transfer the prawns to a bowl and combine with the shallots and coriander.

5   To make the dipping sauce, combine all the ingredients in a small bowl and stir together.

6   Serve the prawns with the lime wedges and dipping sauce.

serves 4

Curried Eggs
with Herb Mayo

I used to love curried egg sandwiches when I was young, so although I don't have the bread these days, I still enjoy the flavour.

8 eggs
2–3 tablespoons Herb Mayo
 (see recipe page 137)
2 teaspoons curry powder
3–4 cornichons, chopped
1 tablespoon capers, rinsed and drained
sea salt and freshly ground black
 pepper, to taste
12 baby cos lettuce leaves

1   Place the eggs in a saucepan and cover with cold water. Bring to the boil then reduce heat to a simmer and cook for 7 minutes. Remove from the heat and run the eggs under cold water, then peel and place in a mixing bowl.

2   Add the herb mayo and curry powder to the eggs and mash with a fork.

3   Add the cornichons and capers, stir to combine, and season with salt and pepper.

4   Serve the curried egg in the lettuce cups.

serves 4

Chicken Schnitzel

The classic schnitty has had a healthy, gluten-free makeover.

4 chicken breast fillets, halved
 horizontally
3 eggs
2 cups arrowroot
2 cups LSA
2 tablespoons fresh thyme leaves
grated zest of 1 lemon
2 tablespoons coconut oil
1 tablespoon butter
sea salt and freshly ground black
 pepper, to taste
2 lemons, cut into segments

1   Using a meat mallet, bash the chicken fillets to 3 mm thickness.

2   In a mixing bowl, whisk the eggs, then add 2 tablespoons of water and lightly whisk together.

3   Place the arrowroot on a large plate. On a separate plate, combine the LSA, thyme and lemon zest.

4   Take each piece of chicken, dip in the arrowroot to coat each side, then dip in the egg mix and lastly dip in the LSA mix. Place the chicken on a baking tray, cover with plastic wrap and chill for 30 minutes.

5   Place a frying pan over medium–high heat and add the coconut oil and butter. Add the chicken (you might need to cook these in two batches) and cook for 5 minutes, or until cooked through and browned on both sides.

6   Season with salt and pepper, and serve with lemon segments alongside.

Curried Eggs with Herb Mayo . 36

Barbecued Banana Prawns with Herb Mayo . 39

serves
4

Zucchini Ribbons with Romesco Sauce

This is a quick and easy recipe, particularly if you have some romesco sauce in the fridge. It works as a snack or side dish, or if you'd like to make it a little more robust, simply add a piece of fried white fish or a can of tuna.

4 large zucchini, cut into ribbons
grated zest of 1 lemon
1 cup black olives, pitted and halved
10 anchovy fillets
2 tablespoons olive oil
⅓ bunch of basil, leaves torn
½ cup Romesco Sauce (see recipe page 134)
sea salt and freshly ground black
  pepper, to taste

1   Bring a saucepan of salted water to the boil. Turn the heat off and add the zucchini. After 10 seconds, remove the zucchini and allow to drain and cool.

2   Place the zucchini in a mixing bowl, add the lemon zest, olives, anchovies and olive oil, and gently toss to combine.

3   Add the torn basil and the romesco sauce, and combine. Season with salt and pepper, and serve.

serves
4

Barbecued Banana Prawns with Herb Mayo

This recipe will work well with Romesco Sauce (see recipe page 134) or even Green Tahini (see recipe page 131). To add a little more tang to the mayo, feel free to add the grated zest of 1 lemon and/or 1 teaspoon of smoked paprika.

24 raw banana prawns
2 tablespoons melted butter
juice of 1 lemon
sea salt and freshly ground black
  pepper, to taste
¼ bunch of coriander, roughly chopped
1 cup Herb Mayo (see recipe page 137)

1   Rinse and drain the prawns then peel, leaving the tails on.

2   Preheat the barbecue to high.

3   Baste the prawns with butter and cook on the barbecue for 1–2 minutes each side, or until the prawns turn pink and opaque.

4   Remove from the heat and dress with lemon juice. Season with salt and pepper, and serve with the coriander and herb mayo alongside.

serves
2

Swordfish with Caper Butter

If you can find Marine Stewardship Council (MSC) certified seafood at your local fishmonger or supermarket, you'll be helping to maintain healthy fish stocks around the world.

2 tablespoons butter
1 garlic clove, chopped or sliced
1 tablespoon baby capers, rinsed and drained
2 swordfish steaks, or other firm white fish such as hoki
sea salt and freshly ground black pepper
¼ bunch fresh dill, chopped, to serve
lemon wedges, to serve

1   Place a frying pan over medium heat and add the butter. Add the garlic and capers and sauté for 1 minute.

2   Add the swordfish and cook for 4–5 minutes each side (time will vary according to thickness of fillets), spooning the butter over the fillets as they cook.

3   Once cooked through, remove the fillets from the heat. Transfer to a serving plate, pour over the caper butter and season to taste. Sprinkle with dill and serve with lemon wedges on the side.

serves
4

20-minute Chicken

This recipe was born because I wanted to use up a few ingredients from a photo shoot and include some chicken I had in the fridge at home. It's very indicative of the sort of food I love – full of flavour, and easy.

2 tablespoons olive oil
1 brown onion, halved and sliced
4 garlic cloves, smashed
500 g chicken thigh fillets, diced
1 teaspoon chilli flakes
1 small punnet of cherry tomatoes
6 anchovy fillets
¼ cup black olives, pitted and halved
sea salt and freshly ground black pepper, to taste

1   Place a large frying pan over low heat and add the olive oil. Add the onion and garlic and sauté for 3–4 minutes.

2   Increase the heat to medium–high and add the chicken, stirring to ensure it is coated in oil. Add the chilli flakes and cook for 5–6 minutes.

3   Reduce the heat to low, add the tomatoes, anchovies and olives and cook for a further 12 minutes, stirring occasionally. Remove from the heat, season with salt and pepper, and serve.

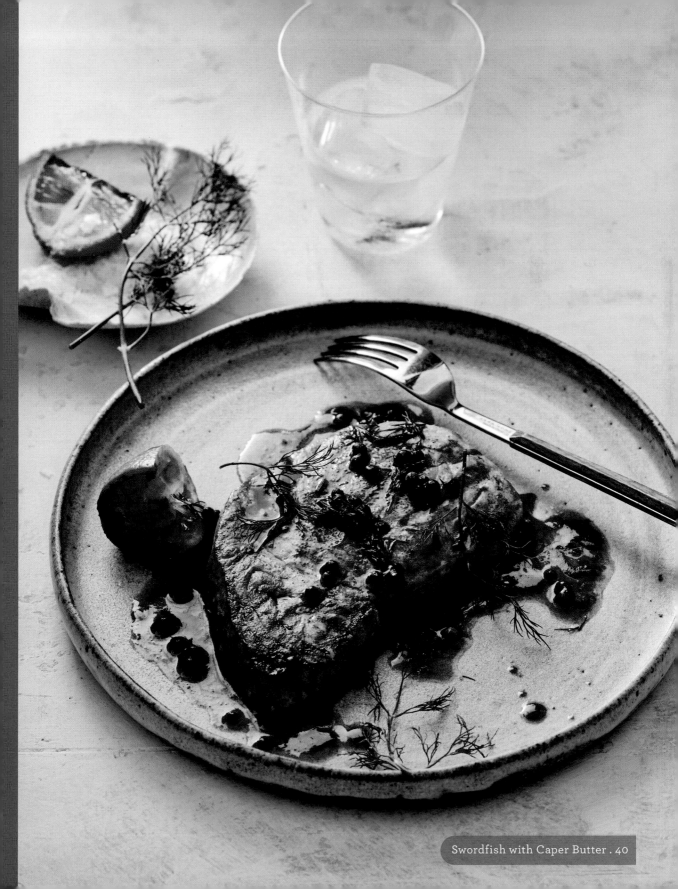

Swordfish with Caper Butter . 40

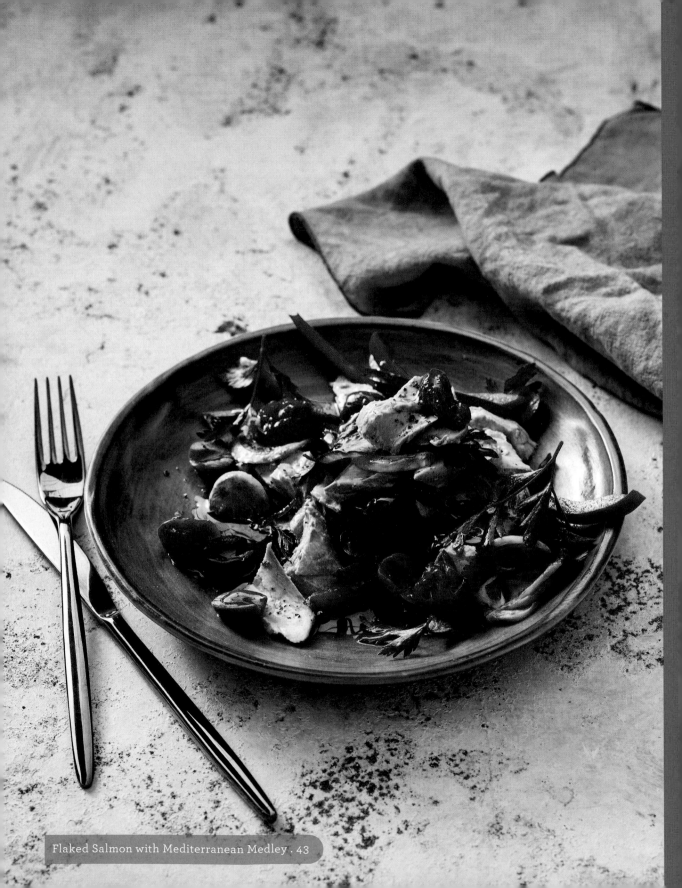

Flaked Salmon with Mediterranean Medley . 43

Flaked Salmon with Mediterranean Medley

This recipe is designed to be fairly loose and rustic. It can be rustled up in less than 15 minutes, but has plenty of flavour and a little sweetness from the capsicum and tomatoes. You can pan-fry the salmon if you'd prefer.

2 tablespoons olive oil
1 onion, chopped
4 garlic cloves, chopped
1 red capsicum, chopped
1 yellow capsicum, chopped
1 green capsicum, chopped
2 baby fennel bulbs, trimmed,
   cored and sliced
1 punnet of cherry tomatoes
3–4 salmon portions
100 g mixed olives, pitted
sea salt and freshly ground black
   pepper, to taste

1   Place a frying pan over low heat and add the olive oil. Add the onion and garlic and sauté for 3–4 minutes.

2   Add the capsicums, fennel and tomatoes and cook for 15 minutes, stirring occasionally.

3   Meanwhile, in a large saucepan, bring some salted water to the boil. Place the salmon in the water, put the lid on and return to the boil, then remove the saucepan from the heat and set aside. After 8–10 minutes, remove the salmon from the water, drain and place in a bowl. Using your fingers, flake the salmon.

4   Add the flaked salmon to the frying pan with the vegetables. Add the olives and cook for a further 4–5 minutes. Remove from the heat, season with salt and pepper, and serve.

Prawn and Egg Tacos

Making your own mayo or aïoli is pretty easy, and I recommend making a big batch and storing it in the fridge. Buying store-bought mayo can be somewhat problematic, as most are made with industralised oils such as canola.

6 eggs
4–5 tablespoons Lime Aïoli
  (see recipe page 134)
½ bunch of dill, finely chopped
1 tablespoon butter
10–12 raw banana prawns, peeled
2 teaspoons baby capers, rinsed
  and drained
12 baby cos lettuce leaves
sea salt and freshly ground black
  pepper, to taste

1 Place the eggs in a small saucepan, cover with cold water and bring to the boil. Reduce the heat to a simmer and cook for 6 minutes (soft boiled). Remove the eggs, run under cold water and peel.

2 In a large mixing bowl, combine the aïoli and eggs and mash together. Add the dill and stir to combine.

3 Place a large frying pan over medium–high heat and add the butter. Add the prawns, gently toss and cook for 3–4 minutes, or until pink and opaque. Remove from the heat and set aside to cool.

4 Once cooled, chop the prawns up and add to the egg mix with the baby capers. Combine thoroughly. Spoon the prawn and egg mix onto each lettuce leaf. Season with salt and pepper, and serve.

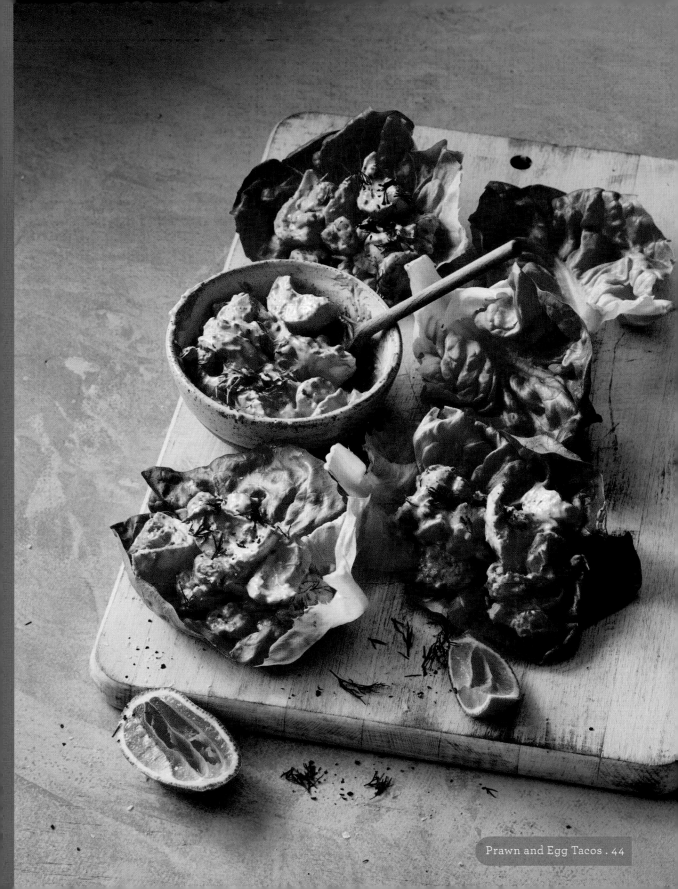

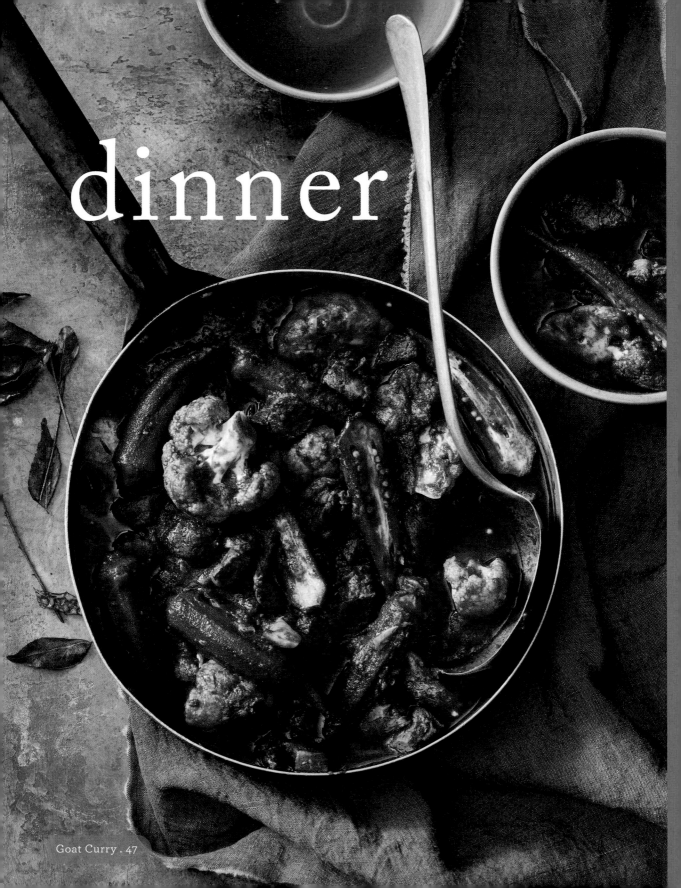

dinner

Goat Curry

If goat isn't available at your local butcher, simply substitute with diced lamb or beef.

500 g diced boneless goat
2 tablespoons ghee
4 red onions, sliced
4 large tomatoes, quartered
500 ml beef bone broth or stock
¼ cauliflower, trimmed and chopped
handful of okra
sea salt and freshly ground black
    pepper, to taste

MARINADE
100 g coconut cream
5 cm knob of ginger, minced
2 garlic cloves, minced
1 teaspoon turmeric
4 teaspoons tomato purée
1 teaspoon garam masala
4 teaspoons Kashmiri chilli paste or
    2 teaspoons Kashmiri chilli powder
sea salt and freshly ground black
    pepper, to taste

1   To make the marinade, place all the ingredients in a large mixing bowl and combine thoroughly.

2   Add the goat meat to the marinade and stir well. Cover and refrigerate for a minimum of 2 hours.

3   Place a large frying pan over medium heat and add the ghee. Add the onion and sauté for 3-4 minutes. Add the tomatoes and cook for a further 3-4 minutes.

4   Add the meat to the pan and cook until the meat is browned, about 8-10 minutes.

5   Add the broth and pop the lid on. Bring to the boil then reduce the heat to low and cook for 40 minutes, stirring occasionally.

6   Add the cauliflower and okra, and cook for a further 15 minutes

7   If the sauce needs reducing, remove the lid and cook until desired consistency is reached. Remove from the heat and allow to rest, uncovered, for 10 minutes. Season with salt and pepper, and serve.

Moules Mariniere

This was one of my favourite dishes as a kid, when my folks ran pubs. I remember my dad leaving an uncovered bucket of NZ green mussels in the cellar – we woke up to them climbing the walls!

2 kg mussels
2 tablespoons butter
2 shallots, trimmed and chopped
2 bay leaves
1 teaspoon dried parsley
1 teaspoon dried thyme
3 garlic cloves, minced
1 cup dry white wine
400 ml coconut cream
¼ bunch of parsley, chopped
sea salt and freshly ground black
    pepper, to taste

1   Rinse the mussels under cold running water, remove any beards and discard all open mussels.

2   Place a large frying pan over low heat and add the butter. Add the shallots, herbs and garlic and sauté for 3–4 minutes.

3   Add the mussels and white wine, turn up the heat to high and pop the lid on. Cook for 3–4 minutes.

4   Add the coconut cream and chopped parsley. Continue to cook for a further 1–2 minutes, or until the shells are open and the mussels cooked. Discard any mussels that don't open.

5   Remove from the heat, season with salt and pepper, and serve.

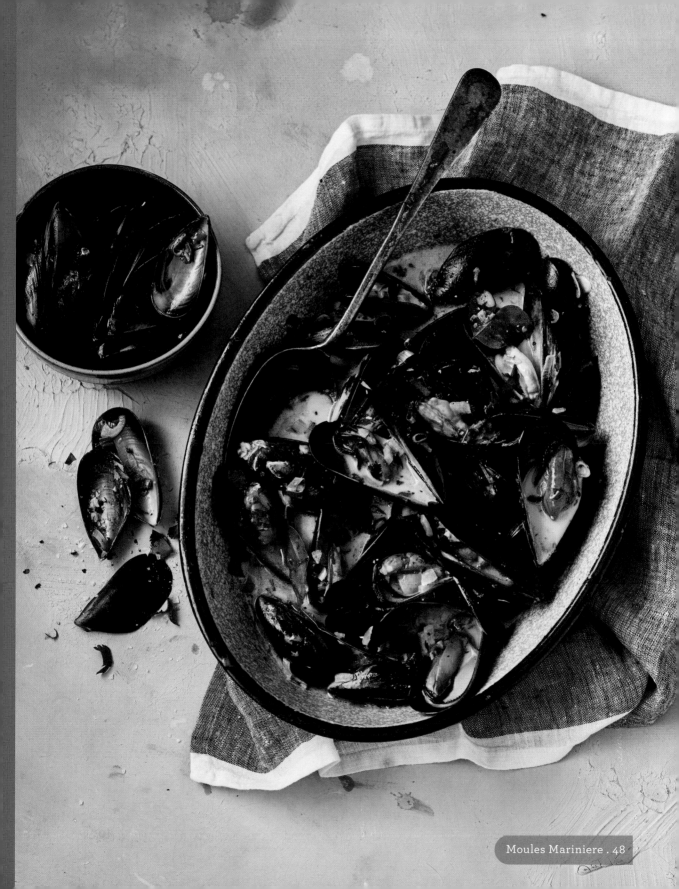

Moules Mariniere . 48

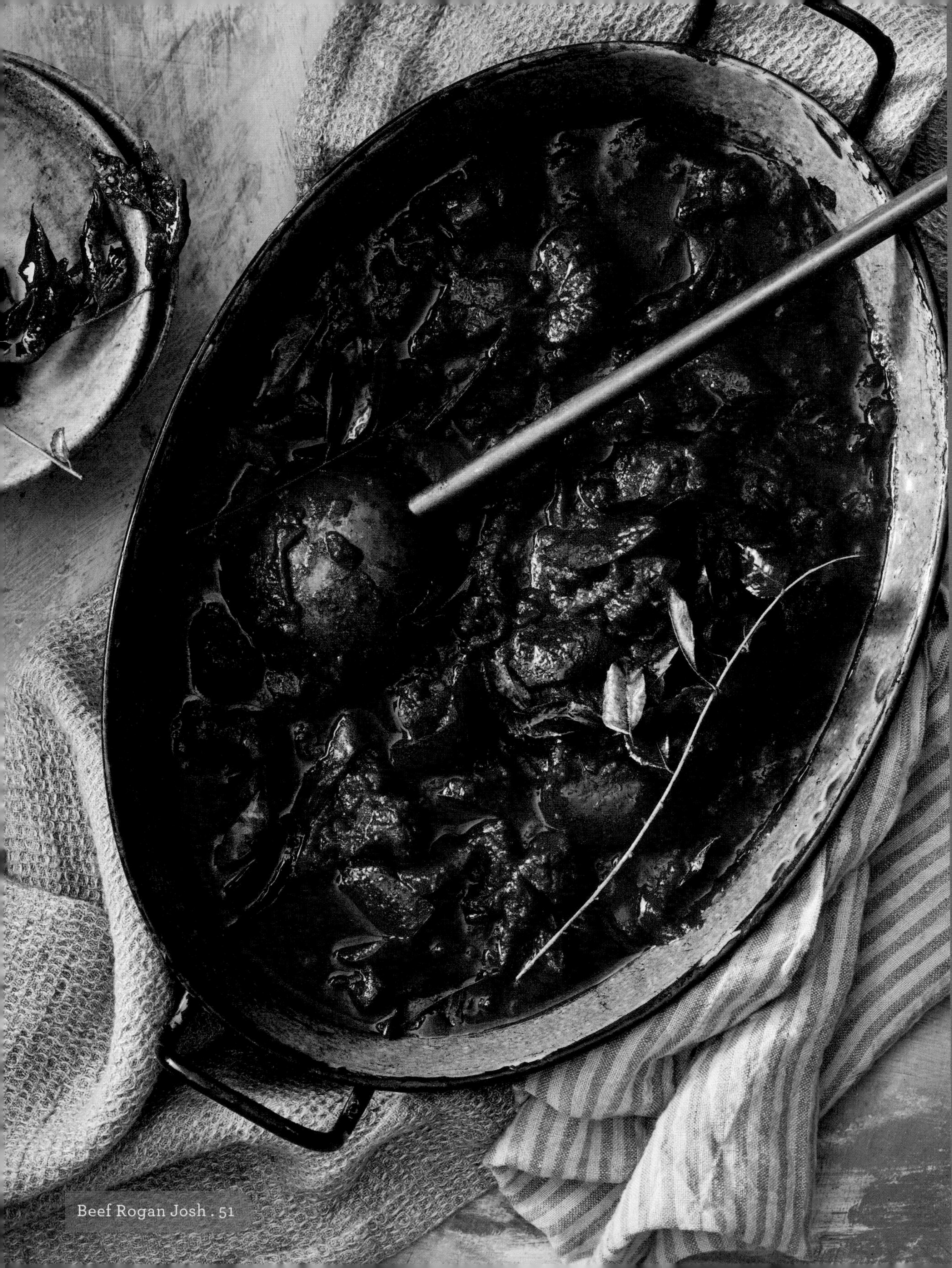

Beef Rogan Josh

I've never met him, but Rogan Josh makes
a damn fine curry. Here's my version.

1 tablespoon ghee
3 red onions, finely chopped
6 garlic cloves, chopped
5 cm knob of ginger, chopped
¼ bunch coriander, stalks removed
    and finely chopped, leaves chopped
4 small red chillies, chopped and
    deseeded (optional)
1 teaspoon cumin
1 tablespoon ground coriander
2 teaspoons paprika
1 tablespoon garam masala
1 teaspoon turmeric
500 g chuck steak, diced
2 red capsicums, deseeded and chopped
1 × 400 g can diced tomatoes
6 ripe tomatoes, quartered
120 ml beef bone broth or stock
sea salt and freshly ground black
    pepper, to taste

1   Place a large saucepan over medium
    heat and add the ghee. Add the onion,
    garlic, ginger, coriander stalks and chilli,
    if using, and sauté for 2–3 minutes. Add
    all the dry spices and stir.

2   Add the beef, stir to ensure it is coated in
    the spice mixture, and cook until browned.

3   Add the capsicum, canned tomatoes,
    fresh tomatoes and broth. Reduce heat to
    low, pop the lid on and cook for 1½ hours,
    stirring occasionally.

4   Remove the lid and simmer to allow curry
    to thicken, about 20 minutes.

5   Remove from the heat, season to taste,
    add chopped coriander leaves and serve.

serves
4

Lamb Tagine

This is a really simple recipe to follow in that
it's 'set and forget'. As long as you don't forget
to take it off the stove, you can't go wrong.

1 tablespoon ghee
2 red onions, finely chopped
2 garlic cloves, finely chopped
1 tablespoon harissa
1 cinnamon stick
1 teaspoon cumin
1 teaspoon ground ginger
1 teaspoon smoked paprika
1 teaspoon sweet paprika
500 g diced lamb leg
2 × 400 g cans diced tomatoes
1 cup beef bone broth or stock
1 bay leaf
2 red capsicums, deseeded and chopped
handful of kalamata olives, pitted and halved
sea salt and freshly ground black pepper,
    to taste

1   Place a large saucepan over medium heat
    and add the ghee. Add the onion and garlic
    and sauté for 2–3 minutes. Add the harissa
    and spices and stir for 1 minute.

2   Add the lamb, stir to ensure it is coated in
    the spice mixture, and cook until browned.

3   Add the tomatoes, broth, bay leaf,
    capsicum and olives. Reduce heat to low,
    pop the lid on and cook for 1½ hours,
    stirring occasionally.

4   Remove the lid and simmer to allow the
    sauce to thicken, about 20 minutes.

5   Remove from the heat, season with salt
    and pepper, and serve.

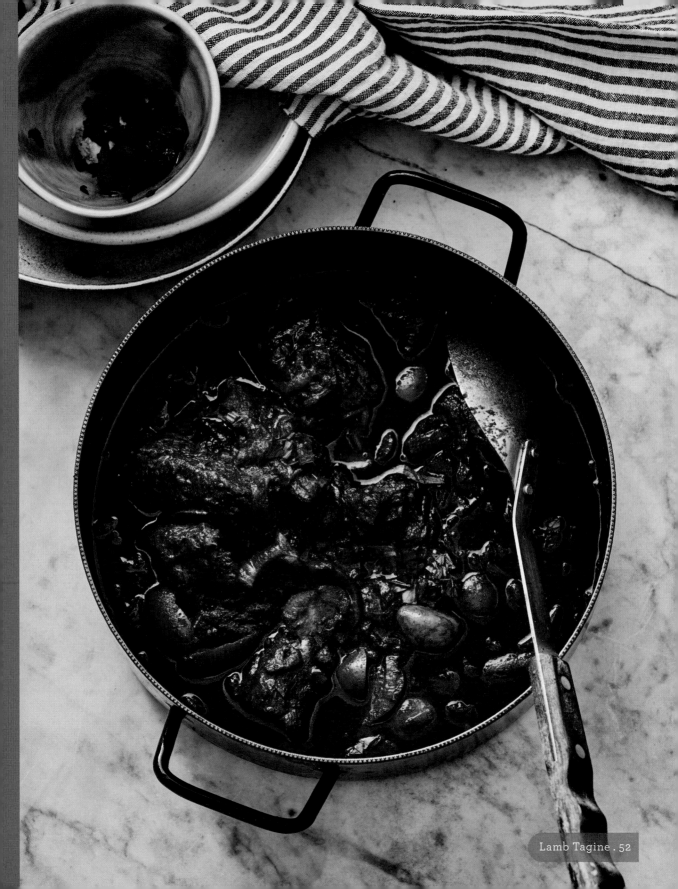

Moroccan Beef Stew . 55

serves
4

Moroccan Beef Stew

This deliciously rich and warming recipe is
guaranteed to get even your mortal enemy
on side!

1 tablespoon ghee
2 onions, finely chopped
6 garlic cloves, finely chopped
1 teaspoon smoked paprika
1 teaspoon sweet paprika
1 tablespoon ras el hanout
2 teaspoons cumin
500 g chuck steak, diced
grated zest of 1 lemon
1 × 400 g can diced tomatoes
500 ml beef bone broth or stock
400 g red or brown lentils
handful of green olives, pitted and halved
sea salt and black pepper, to taste

1   Place a large saucepan over medium heat
    and add the ghee. Add the onion and garlic
    and sauté for 2–3 minutes. Add the spices
    and stir to combine.

2   Increase the heat, add the beef and cook
    until brown all over.

3   Add the lemon zest, tomato, broth, lentils
    and olives. Reduce heat to low, pop the
    lid on and cook for 1½ hours, stirring
    occasionally.

4   Remove the lid and simmer to allow the
    sauce to thicken, about 20 minutes.

5   Remove from the heat, and season with
    salt and pepper before serving.

serves
2

serves
4

Rump Steak with Anchovy Butter

I'm salivating just thinking about this dish ...!

2 rump steaks
1 tablespoon olive oil
sea salt and freshly ground black
   pepper, to taste
2 tablespoons Anchovy Butter
   (see recipe page 136)

1   Remove the steaks from the fridge
    30 minutes prior to cooking.

2   Place a frying pan over high heat and
    add the oil. Season both sides of the steak
    with salt and pepper and place in the pan.
    Depending on the thickness of the steak,
    cook for 2–3 minutes on each side. Once
    cooked to your liking, remove from the
    heat and allow to rest for 2 minutes.

3   Spoon 1 tablespoon of anchovy butter
    on top of each steak before serving.

Chilli Salt Scotch Fillet with Chimichurri

There are a couple of heroes in this dish, but
it's really all about the dressing – the acidity
of the chimichurri is great with steak,
particularly fatty cuts.

3 garlic cloves, minced
½ teaspoon chilli flakes
1 teaspoon dried oregano
1 tablespoon coconut oil
4 grass-fed Scotch fillets
sea salt and freshly ground black
   pepper, to taste
1 teaspoon ghee
1 cup Chimichurri (see recipe page 130)

1   Using a pestle and mortar, or in a mixing
    bowl, combine the garlic, chilli flakes,
    oregano and coconut oil. Rub the marinade
    into the steak, season with salt and pepper,
    and set aside.

2   Place a frying pan over high heat and
    add the ghee. Add the steaks (perhaps
    do two at a time, or heat two pans).
    Cook for 3 minutes on each side for rare.
    Remove from the heat and allow to rest
    for 2–3 minutes.

3   Serve the steak with the chimichurri.

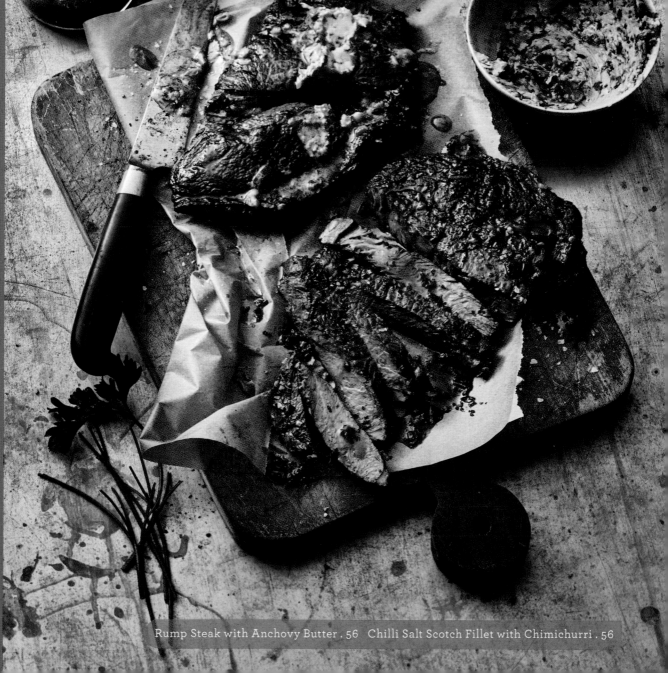

Rump Steak with Anchovy Butter . 56   Chilli Salt Scotch Fillet with Chimichurri . 56

Spanish Oxtail Stew

I remember peering into a large, simmering pot on the stovetop as a kid and asking my dad what was in there. 'Oxtail, son, oxtail!' he replied. I've been eating oxtail ever since.

2 tablespoons olive oil
2 kg oxtail, cut into 5 cm pieces
    (ask the butcher to do this for you)
2 gluten-free chorizo, roughly chopped
1 onion, chopped
4 garlic cloves, chopped
1 tablespoon smoked paprika
1 teaspoon sweet paprika
1 teaspoon dried oregano
6 sprigs of rosemary
2 medium carrots, sliced
240 ml dry white wine
500 ml chicken broth or stock
2 × 400 g cans diced tomatoes
sea salt and freshly ground black
    pepper, to taste
¼ bunch of parsley, roughly chopped

1   Preheat your oven to 150°C.

2   Place a lidded casserole or ovenproof dish over high heat and heat 1 tablespoon of the olive oil. Add the oxtail (you may have to do this in batches) and cook until all the pieces are browned off. Remove and set aside.

3   Add the chorizo to the pan and fry until caramelised, then set aside.

4   Add the remaining olive oil to the dish and reduce the heat to medium. Add the onion and garlic and sauté for 3–4 minutes.

5   Add the paprika, oregano, rosemary and carrot and cook for 1–2 minutes.

6   Add the white wine, increase heat to high and cook for 1–2 minutes, or until the alcohol is evaporated. Add the broth.

7   Place the oxtail and chorizo in the dish, add the tomatoes, and season with salt and pepper. Pop the lid on and bake for 3–3½ hours, or until the meat is tender and falls off the bone. Remove from the oven and allow to rest for 15 minutes.

8   Before serving, add the chopped parsley, and season again with salt and pepper if needed.

serves
4+

Hoki Bouillabaisse

This dish is a real show-stopper when placed on the dinner table – a great dish to serve up when the in-laws are over.

12 mussels
2 tablespoons olive oil
3 garlic cloves, chopped
1 brown onion, diced
1 fennel bulb, trimmed, cored
    and diced
1 carrot, diced
½ teaspoon saffron
1 teaspoon fennel seeds
1 teaspoon dried thyme
2 bay leaves
240 ml white wine
500 ml fish stock
2 × 400 g cans diced tomatoes
400 g hoki fillets, skin removed,
    chopped
6 raw banana prawns, peeled and
    deveined
sea salt and freshly ground black
    pepper, to taste
6 basil leaves, torn

1   Rinse the mussels under cold running water, remove any beards and discard all open mussels. Set aside.

2   Place a large saucepan over medium heat and add the olive oil. Add the garlic, onion, fennel and carrot and allow to sweat for 3–4 minutes, stirring occasionally. Add the herbs and spices and cook for a further 1 minute.

3   Increase the heat to high, add the white wine and cook for 1–2 minutes, or until the alcohol is evaporated.

4   Add the fish stock and tomatoes and bring to the boil, then reduce heat to low. Allow to simmer for 15 minutes.

5   Add the fish and cook for 5–6 minutes, or until cooked through and opaque.

6   With 3–4 minutes of cooking time remaining, add the prawns and mussels.

7   Once the prawns and mussels have cooked, remove the pan from the heat. Season with salt and pepper, throw in the basil, and serve.

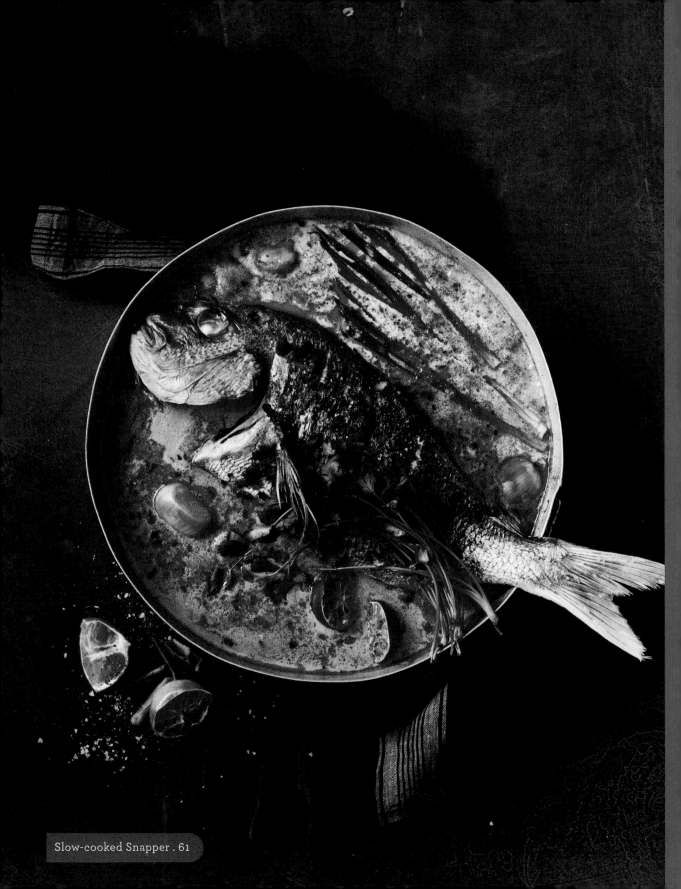

serves
4

Slow-cooked Snapper

My love for slow-cooked dishes runs deep
and includes whole fish. As you can see,
the end result is quite stunning.

1 tablespoon coconut oil
1 brown onion, finely chopped
2 shallots, trimmed and chopped
5 cm knob of ginger, minced
4 garlic cloves, minced
3 tablespoons curry powder
4 eschalots, peeled
400 ml coconut milk (or more if needed)
flesh of 1 young coconut, chopped (optional)
2 tablespoons fish sauce
juice of 1 lime
1 teaspoon honey
1 whole snapper (approx. 700 g)
sea salt and freshly ground black pepper,
    to taste
¼ bunch of coriander, roughly chopped

1   Preheat your oven to 140°C.

2   Place a frying pan over medium heat
    and add the coconut oil. Add the onion,
    shallots, ginger, garlic, curry powder and
    eschalots. Sauté for 4–5 minutes, or until
    the vegetables have taken up the colour
    of the curry powder. Remove from the
    heat and set aside to cool.

3   In a lidded casserole or baking dish big
    enough for the fish, combine the coconut
    milk, coconut flesh if using, fish sauce,
    lime juice and honey.

4   Make 3–4 incisions on the snapper,
    cutting deep enough to hit the backbone.
    Using your fingers, rub the cooled onion
    mixture into the incisions. Place the fish in
    the baking dish. The liquid should cover at
    least 80 per cent the fish; add more coconut
    milk if needed. Pop the lid on and bake for
    1½ hours.

5   Remove from the oven and season
    with salt and pepper. Add the chopped
    coriander before serving.

Jerk Chicken

1½ tablespoons allspice
2 cm knob of ginger, roughly chopped
2 teaspoons cinnamon
3 garlic cloves, halved
2 hot habaneros chillies, deseeded
2 tablespoons honey
3 shallots, trimmed and roughly chopped
1 tablespoon dried thyme
4 tablespoons lime juice
2 tablespoons olive oil
500 g chicken thigh or breast fillets
¼ bunch of coriander, roughly chopped
sea salt, to taste

1 Combine all the ingredients except the chicken and coriander in a blender or food processor and blitz for 20 seconds. Transfer to a mixing bowl, add the chicken and coat the chicken well. Marinate in the fridge for 2 hours.

2 Preheat your oven to 180°C.

3 Line a baking tray with baking paper. Tip the chicken onto the tray and bake for 40–45 minutes, or until golden and cooked through. Garnish with coriander and season again with salt if needed.

Beef Goulash

I can still recall the smells wafting up the stairs as a kid when Mum was cooking up the daily specials for the pub. Goulash was one of the dishes that was unmistakable, and a real treat when I got home from school.

1 tablespoon ghee
2 brown onions, roughly chopped
2 garlic cloves, roughly chopped
500 g chuck steak, diced
1 large red capsicum, sliced
3 carrots, diced
1 × 400 g can diced tomatoes
200 ml tomato passata
500 ml beef bone broth or stock
2 tablespoons sweet paprika
2 teaspoons caraway seeds
1 bay leaf
sea salt and freshly ground black pepper, to taste
½ bunch of parsley, roughly chopped

1 Place a large, lidded frying pan or saucepan over medium heat and add the ghee. Add the onion and garlic and sauté for 4–5 minutes, or until softened.

2 Increase the heat to high, add the steak and cook until browned.

3 Add all the remaining ingredients except the parsley.

4 Reduce the heat to low, pop the lid on the pan and cook for 1½ hours, or until the beef is tender. Remove the lid and continue simmering to thicken the sauce to your desired consistency.

5 Remove from the heat, and scatter with parsley before serving.

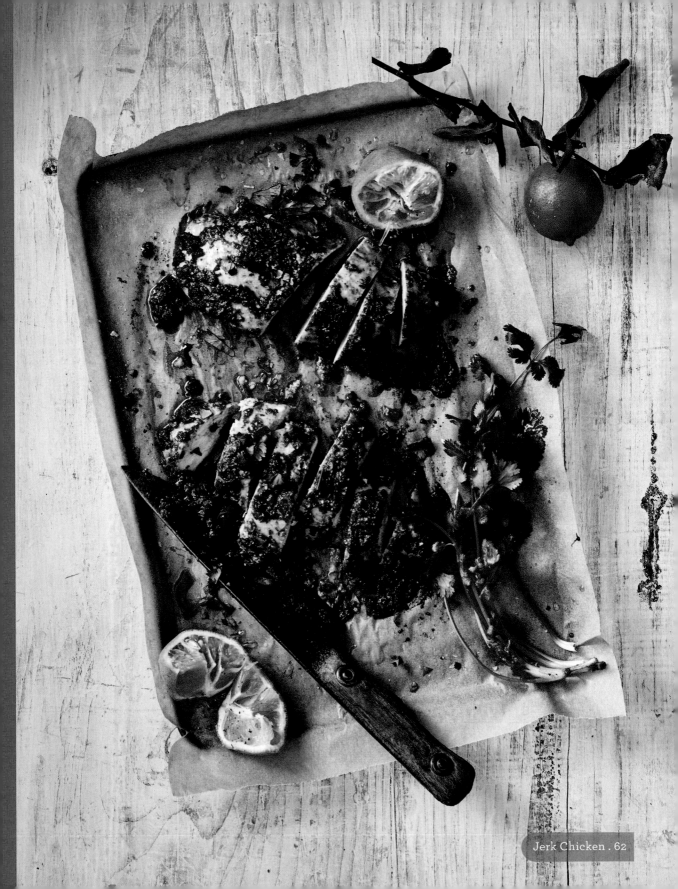

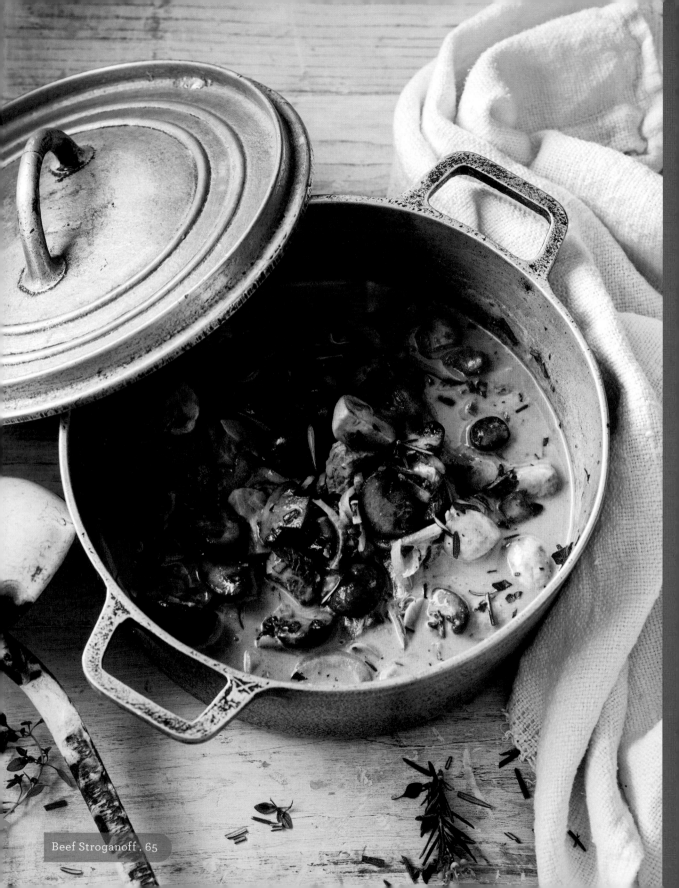

Beef Stroganoff . 65

Beef Stroganoff

2 tablespoons ghee
1 onion, chopped
2 garlic cloves, chopped
500 g beef tenderloins or rump,
    cut into strips
½ cup white wine
1 cup beef bone broth or stock
1 tablespoon dried thyme
1 tablespoon dried rosemary
3 teaspoons Dijon mustard
400 ml coconut cream
large handful of button mushrooms, halved
sea salt and freshly ground pepper,
    to taste

1   Place a large saucepan over medium
    heat and add the ghee. Add the onion
    and garlic and sauté for 2–3 minutes.

2   Add the beef and cook until browned
    all over.

3   Add the wine and cook until the alcohol
    is evaporated, about 1 minute. Add the
    broth, herbs and mustard and stir.

4   Add the coconut cream. Add the
    mushrooms and cook for 7–8 minutes,
    or until just cooked.

5   Season with salt and pepper, and serve.

Barbecued Herb Butter Prawns

A perfect addition to a summer barbecue.

120 g salted butter
3 garlic cloves, minced
1 long red chilli, deseeded and
    roughly chopped
½ bunch of parsley, chopped
24 raw banana prawns
juice of 1 lemon
sea salt and freshly ground black
    pepper, to taste

1   Preheat the barbecue to medium.

2   Place a frying pan over low–medium heat
    and add the butter. Cook for 2 minutes,
    then add the garlic and chilli and cook for
    a further 2 minutes. Add the parsley and
    cook for a further 1 minute. Remove the
    pan from the heat but keep warm.

3   Throw the prawns on the barbecue.
    Using a brush, smear some of the butter
    from the pan onto the prawns as they cook,
    ensuring both sides are covered. Cook
    for 1–2 minutes each side, or until cooked
    through.

4   Remove the prawns from the barbecue
    and coat with more of the herb butter and
    a drizzle of lemon juice. Season with salt
    and pepper, and serve.

Beef Madras

For years, Indian cuisine was considered
unhealthy, but authentic Indian food is
full of healthful ingredients such as spices,
ghee and coconut milk.

1 tablespoon ghee
2 small brown onions, roughly chopped
4 garlic cloves, roughly chopped
2 red chillies, deseeded and roughly
   chopped
2 tablespoons ground coriander
1 tablespoon cumin
1 teaspoon turmeric
1 teaspoon ground chilli
500 g chuck steak, diced
1 cup tomato passata
450 ml beef bone broth or stock
100 ml coconut cream
½ bunch of coriander, roughly chopped
sea salt and freshly ground black pepper,
   to taste
Honorine's Coconut Sambal
   (see recipe page 124), to serve (optional)

1   Place a deep saucepan over medium heat
    and add the ghee. Add the onion, garlic
    and chilli and sauté for 2–3 minutes. Add
    the spices and stir for 1 minute.

2   Add the beef, stir to coat with the spice
    mixture and cook until the beef is browned.

3   Add the tomato passata, broth and coconut
    cream. Pop the lid on and reduce the heat
    to low. Simmer for 1½ hours, or until the
    beef is tender, stirring occasionally during
    the cooking process.

4   To thicken the sauce, remove the lid and
    increase the heat. Alternatively, if the curry
    is too thick, add some water. Remove from
    the heat, season and garnish with chopped
    coriander before serving with coconut
    sambal, if desired.

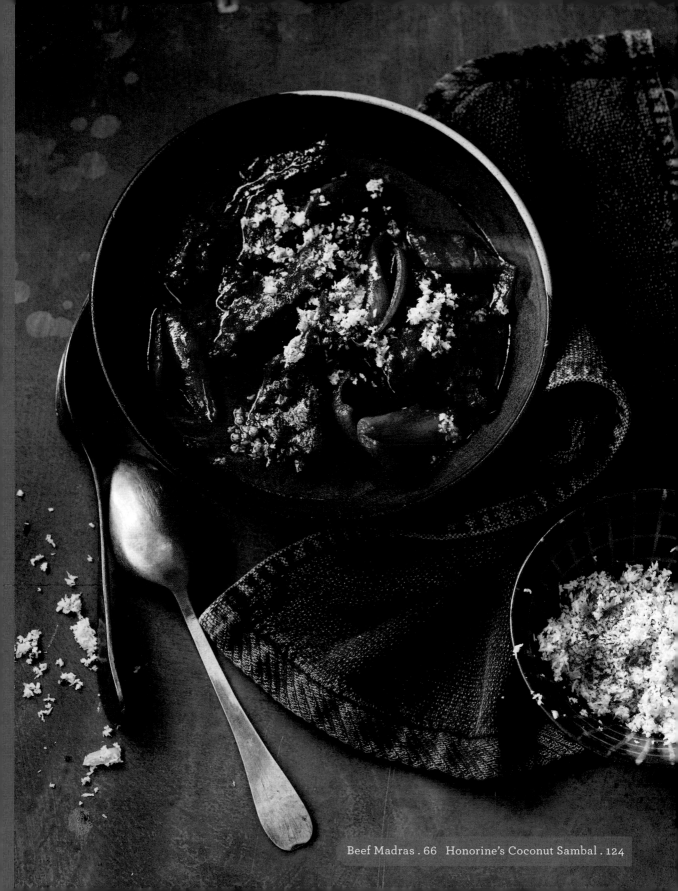

Beef Madras . 66   Honorine's Coconut Sambal . 124

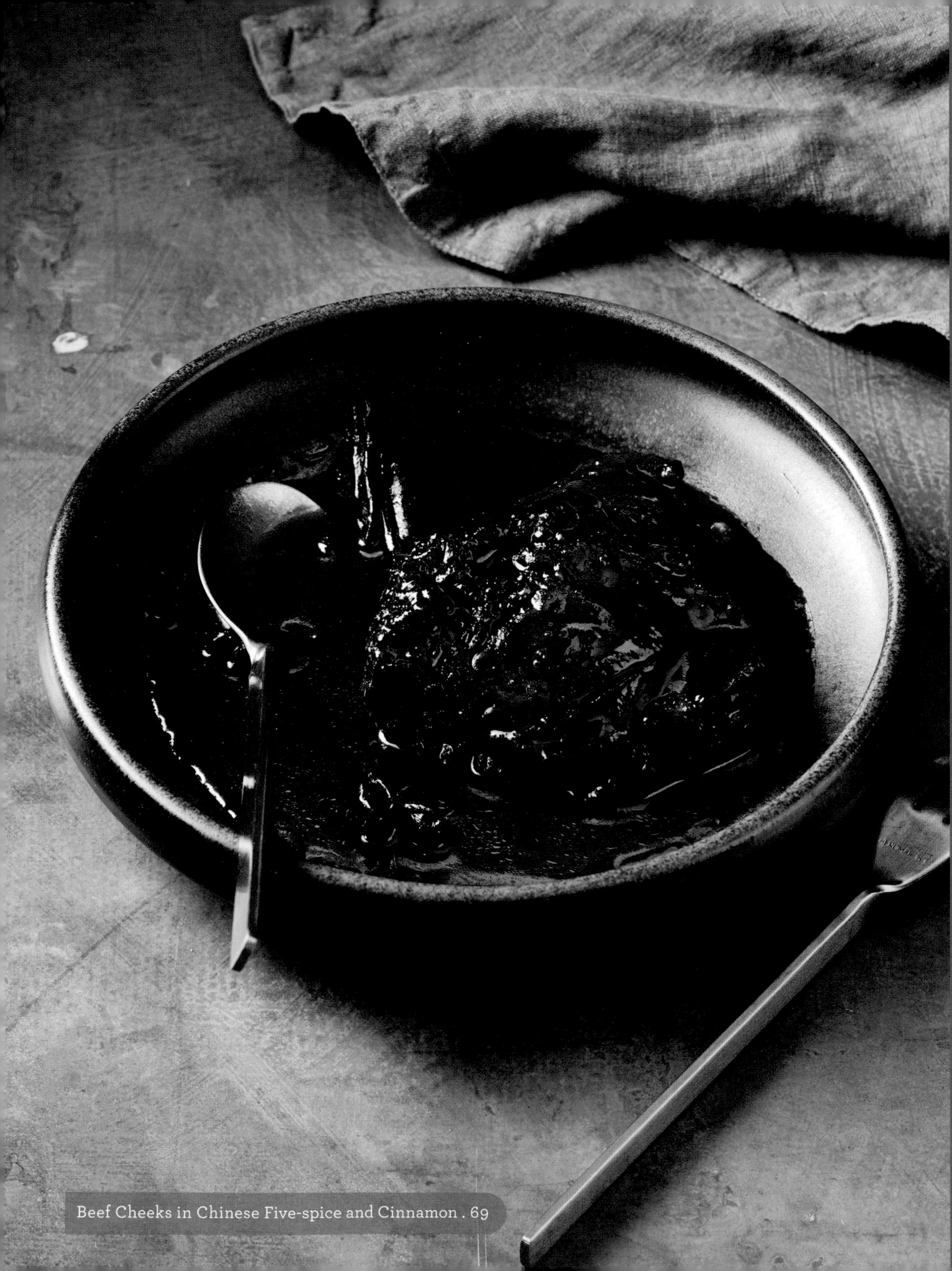

Beef Cheeks in Chinese Five-spice and Cinnamon . 69

serves
4-6

Beef Cheeks in Chinese Five-spice and Cinnamon

If I had to pick a dish to eat for the rest of my life then this would be it. Once you reduce the broth you'll understand why.

1 tablespoon ghee
3–4 beef cheeks
2 cinnamon sticks
2 star anise
2 teaspoons Chinese five-spice
2 tablespoons honey
4 small brown onions, quartered
4 garlic cloves, quartered
1 litre beef bone broth or stock
sea salt and freshly ground black
  pepper, to taste

1   Preheat your oven to 250°C.

2   Place a large frying pan over high heat and add the ghee. Add the beef cheeks and cook until browned all over. Remove from the heat and place in a lidded casserole or ovenproof dish.

3   Add the remaining ingredients, adding water if necessary (the cheeks should be 90 per cent covered with liquid). Pop the lid on and place in the oven. Reduce the oven temperature to 140°C and cook for 4 hours, or until the cheeks fall apart.

4   Drain the liquid from the casserole dish into your frying pan and rapidly reduce over high heat. Once the sauce is reduced, remove from the heat, season with salt and pepper, and serve with the beef cheeks.

serves
6

Pulled Lamb with Reduction

I'm not a chef, but if I was this would be my signature dish – it's the best!

6 sprigs of rosemary
6 sprigs of thyme
1.5 kg shoulder of lamb (on the bone)
2 tablespoons caraway seeds
4 brown onions, quartered
6 garlic cloves, halved
1 litre beef bone broth or stock
  (or more if needed)
sea salt and freshly ground black
  pepper, to taste

1   Preheat your oven to 250°C.

2   Select a lidded casserole or ovenproof dish, place the herb sprigs on the bottom and place the lamb shoulder on top. Sprinkle over the caraway seeds and scatter the onion and garlic around the lamb.

3   Pour the broth into the dish. The liquid should cover 80 per cent of the lamb; add more water or broth if needed. Season with salt and pepper, pop the lid on and place in the oven. Reduce the temperature to 140°C and cook for 6 hours.

4   Remove from the oven and drain the liquid from the dish into a large frying pan. Place the frying pan over high heat and reduce to a richer, thicker jus. Pour the reduction back onto the lamb before serving.

serves
4

Chicken Peri Peri

The combination of tang, spices, fat and salt make this dish quite irresistible.

3 tablespoons ghee or olive oil
juice of ½ lemon
2 teaspoons chilli flakes
3 garlic cloves, finely chopped
4 cm knob of ginger, finely chopped
2 teaspoons sweet paprika
¼ teaspoon cayenne pepper
1 teaspoon dried oregano
sea salt and freshly ground black
   pepper, to taste
500 g chicken thigh fillets
lime halves, to serve

1   In a small food processor, blitz all the ingredients except the chicken to a smooth paste.

2   Combine the paste with the chicken in a large mixing bowl and marinate for a minimum of 30 minutes in the fridge.

3   Preheat your oven to 180°C.

4   Transfer the chicken to a baking tray and bake for 20 minutes, then increase the temperature to 220°C and bake for a further 15 minutes, or until the chicken is cooked through and golden. Season if desired and serve with lime halves.

serves
4

Chicken and Pumpkin Curry

1 tablespoon coconut oil
2 garlic cloves, finely chopped
3 teaspoons Thai seven-spice
5 cm knob of ginger, minced
1 stalk of lemongrass, white part only,
   thinly sliced
1–2 bird's-eye chillies, finely chopped
500 g chicken thigh fillets, chopped
¼ butternut pumpkin, peeled and chopped
¼ cauliflower, cut into small florets
½ red capsicum, deseeded and chopped
½ green capsicum, deseeded and chopped
1 × 400 ml can coconut cream
200 ml vegetable or chicken stock
1 teaspoon tamarind paste
⅓ bunch of English spinach, roughly chopped
¼ bunch of coriander, chopped

1   Place a large saucepan over medium heat and add the coconut oil. Add the garlic, seven-spice, ginger, lemongrass and chilli and sauté for 3–4 minutes.

2   Add the chicken and cook, stirring, for a further 3–4 minutes.

3   Add the pumpkin, cauliflower and capsicum, toss well and cook for 2–3 minutes. Add the coconut cream and stock and cook for 15–20 minutes, or until the chicken is cooked through and the sauce is thickened to your liking.

4   Add the tamarind and spinach, stir through and cook for 1–2 minutes, or until the spinach has softened.

5   Remove from the heat. Before serving, add the coriander and stir through.

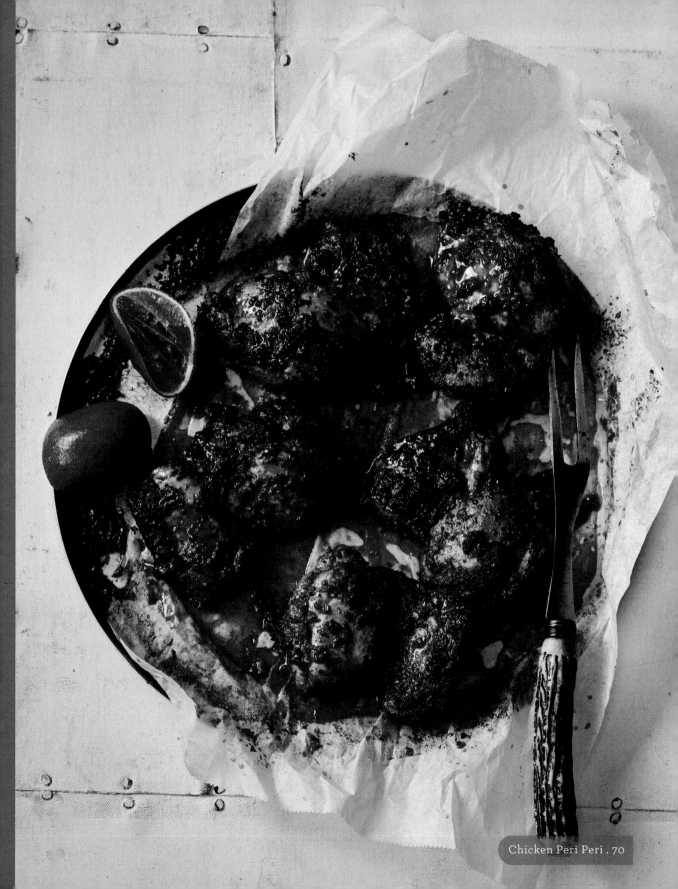

Chicken Peri Peri . 70

Coconut and Pumpkin Curry . 73

Coconut and Pumpkin Curry

1 tablespoon coconut oil
2 garlic cloves, finely chopped
3 teaspoons Thai seven-spice
2 cm knob of ginger, minced
1 stalk of lemongrass, white part only,
   thinly sliced
1–2 bird's-eye chillies, finely chopped
¼ butternut pumpkin, peeled and chopped
¼ cauliflower, cut into small florets
½ red capsicum, deseeded and chopped
¼ green capsicum, deseeded and chopped
1 × 400 ml can coconut cream
1 cup vegetable stock
1 teaspoon tamarind paste
⅓ bunch of English spinach, roughly
   chopped
¼ bunch of coriander, chopped

1   Place a large saucepan over medium heat
    and add the coconut oil. Add the garlic,
    seven-spice, ginger, lemongrass and chilli
    and sauté for 4–5 minutes.

2   Add the pumpkin, cauliflower and capsicum,
    toss well and cook for 2–3 minutes. Add
    the coconut cream and stock and cook
    for 15–20 minutes, or until the pumpkin is
    cooked through and the sauce is thickened
    to your liking.

3   Add the tamarind and spinach, stir through
    and cook for 1–2 minutes, or until the
    spinach has softened.

4   Remove from the heat. Before serving,
    add the coriander and stir through.

serves
2

Vegetarian Korma

This korma recipe is a delicious dish for anyone new to Indian cuisine. Much like butter chicken, it's mild, creamy and yummy.

1 tablespoon coconut oil
1 brown onion, finely chopped
1 teaspoon ground cardamom
2 teaspoons cumin
2 teaspoons ground coriander
½ teaspoon turmeric
1 green chilli, deseeded and finely chopped
5 cm knob of ginger, minced
1 zucchini, sliced
¼ pumpkin, peeled and chopped
¼ head of cauliflower, cut into florets
350 ml vegetable stock
1 × 400 ml can coconut cream
sea salt and freshly ground black pepper,
   to taste
¼ cup almond flakes, toasted

1   Place a large saucepan over low heat and add the coconut oil. Add the onion and dried spices and sauté for 3–4 minutes.

2   Add the chilli and ginger and cook for 2–3 minutes.

3   Add the zucchini, pumpkin and cauliflower and stir to ensure the vegetables are coated in spices. Cook for a further 5 minutes.

4   Add the stock and coconut cream and continue to cook until the sauce reduces to your desired consistency.

5   Remove from the heat and season with salt and pepper. Before serving, garnish with toasted almond flakes.

serves
4

Chicken Korma

1 tablespoon coconut oil
1 brown onion, finely chopped
1 teaspoon ground cardamom
2 teaspoons cumin
2 teaspoons ground coriander
½ teaspoon turmeric
500 g chicken thigh fillets, chopped
1 green chilli, deseeded and finely chopped
5 cm knob of ginger, minced
1 zucchini, sliced
¼ pumpkin, peeled and chopped
¼ head of cauliflower, cut into florets
350 ml vegetable stock
400 ml coconut cream
sea salt and freshly ground black pepper,
   to taste
¼ cup almond flakes, toasted

1   Place a large saucepan over low heat and add the coconut oil. Add the onion and dried spices and sauté for 3–4 minutes.

2   Add the chicken, increase the temperature to medium–high and cook for 3–4 minutes.

3   Add the chilli and ginger and cook for 2–3 minutes.

4   Add the zucchini, pumpkin and cauliflower and stir to ensure the vegetables are coated in spices. Cook for a further 5 minutes.

5   Add the stock and coconut cream and continue to cook until the sauce reduces to your desired consistency.

6   Remove from the heat and season with salt and pepper. Before serving, garnish with toasted almond flakes.

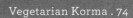

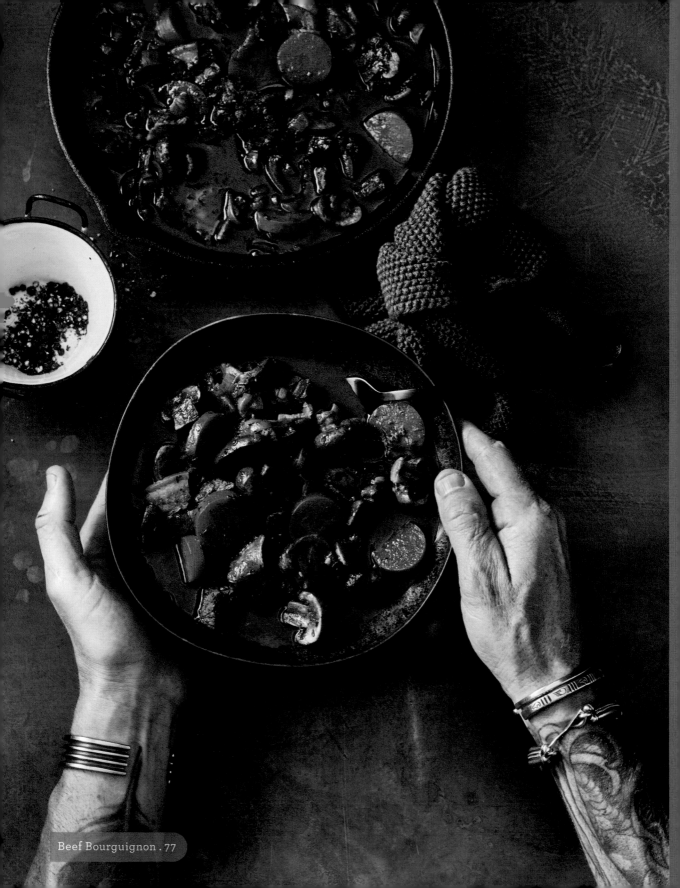

Beef Bourguignon . 77

serves
4

Beef Bourguignon

Make a big batch of this rich and delicious dish and store it in the fridge or freezer for when you're pressed for time.

1 tablespoon olive oil
150 g bacon, chopped
2 onions, chopped
4 garlic cloves, chopped
2 bay leaves
2 teaspoons dried thyme
1 teaspoon dried sage
500 g chuck steak, diced
2 carrots, sliced
250 ml red wine
750 ml beef bone broth or stock
   (or more if needed)
200 g button mushrooms, halved
sea salt and freshly ground black
   pepper, to taste

1 Place a large saucepan over medium heat and add the olive oil. Add the bacon and cook until browned and the fat has rendered. Remove from the saucepan and set aside.

2 Add the onion and garlic and sauté for 3–4 minutes. Add the herbs and cook for 1 minute.

3 Add the diced beef and stir to coat with herbs and onion. Cook for 5–6 minutes, or until the beef is browned.

4 Add the carrot and cook for 1 minute.

5 Add the red wine and cook for 1–2 minutes over high heat until the alcohol has evaporated, then add the broth and bring to the boil. Once boiling, reduce the heat to low and simmer for 1½ hours (add more broth or water if you need to).

6 With 10 minutes of cooking time to go, add the cooked bacon and the mushrooms.

7 Remove from the heat and season with salt and pepper.

Chicken Saagwala

This a really easy recipe and is a superb way
to get a good hit of greens in for the day.

2 tablespoons ghee
1 onion, sliced
4 garlic cloves, chopped
2 cm knob of ginger, minced
1 tablespoon mild curry powder
2 teaspoons cumin seeds
2 teaspoons ground coriander
1 bunch of English spinach, trimmed
    and roughly chopped
100 g coconut yoghurt
500 g chicken thigh fillets, chopped
sea salt and freshly ground black
    pepper, to taste
lemon wedges, to serve

1   Place a large frying pan over medium
    heat and add 1 tablespoon of the ghee.
    Add the onion, garlic and ginger and sauté
    for 3–4 minutes. Add the curry powder,
    cumin and coriander and cook, stirring,
    for 1–2 minutes. Remove from the heat
    and set aside.

2   In a saucepan, bring some salted water to
    the boil. Add the spinach for 20 seconds to
    blanch. Remove from the water and drain.

3   Place the spinach in a food processor
    or blender, add the onion mixture and
    yoghurt and blitz for 20–30 seconds.

4   Place your large frying pan over medium-
    high heat and add the remaining ghee.
    Add the chicken and cook, stirring, for
    5–6 minutes.

5   Add the spinach sauce, stir and continue
    to cook for a further 5–6 minutes, or until
    the chicken is cooked through.

6   Remove from the heat, season with salt
    and pepper and serve with lemon wedges.

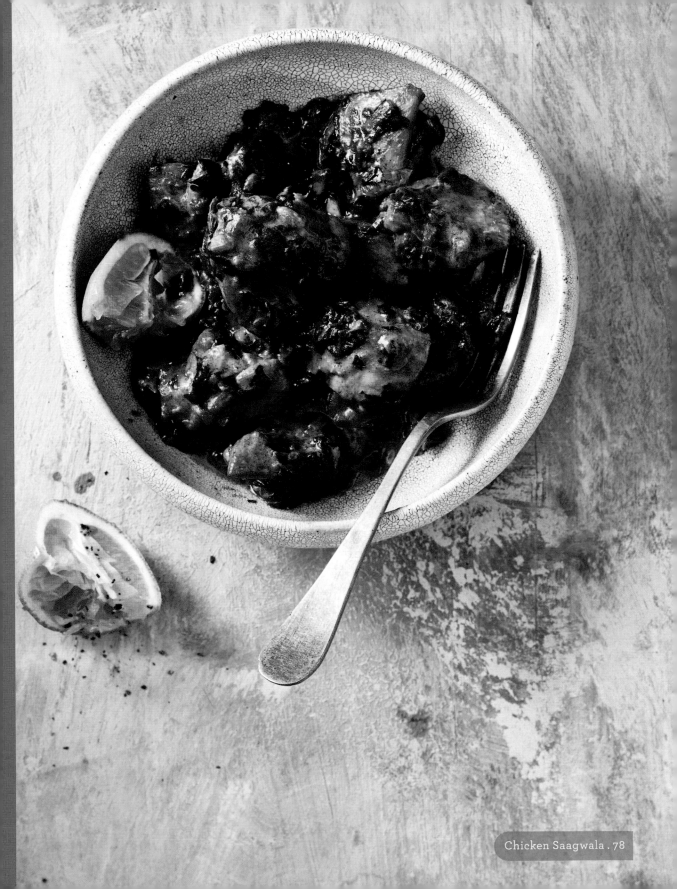

Chicken Saagwala . 78

Side of Salmon with Tahini Dressing . 81

Side of Salmon with Tahini Dressing

If you're having a few friends over for lunch, this dish looks decadent and fancy but it's actually really simple, taking only 20 minutes to make. Once the salmon is cooking, throw together the tahini dressing and extract the pomegranate seeds and you'll be set to dress the fish once it's ready.

1 fillet of salmon (1 whole side)
1 tablespoon olive oil
¼ bunch of dill, roughly chopped
⅓ cup crushed pistachios
¼ cup pomegranate seeds
juice of 1 lemon
2 tablespoons walnut or olive oil
4–5 tablespoons Tahini Dressing
   (see recipe page 131)
sea salt and freshly ground black
   pepper, to taste

1   Preheat your oven to 180°C.

2   Line a large baking tray (long enough to hold the fish) with baking paper. Place the fish on the tray. Drizzle a little olive oil over the fish. Bake for 20 minutes for rare, or until cooked to your liking. Remove from the oven and allow to rest for 5 minutes.

3   In a bowl, gently toss together the dill, pistachios and pomegranate seeds. Scatter the mixture over the fish and drizzle the fish with the lemon juice, walnut oil and tahini. Season with salt and pepper, and serve.

serves
4

Red Chicken Curry

A Thai curry is on the money for flavour
and health, I reckon. Full of veggies and spice,
not to mention healthy fats, this recipe is a
family favourite.

1 tablespoon coconut oil
2 shallots, trimmed and chopped
2–3 tablespoons red curry paste (see below)
500 g chicken thigh fillets, chopped
2 cups chopped peeled pumpkin
75 g sugar snap peas
1 × 400 ml can coconut milk
sea salt and freshly ground black pepper,
    to taste
¼ bunch of coriander, leaves chopped,
    to garnish
lime wedges, to serve

RED CURRY PASTE
8 dried red chillies, soaked in water for
    10 minutes
10 garlic cloves
1 stalk of lemongrass, white part only,
    chopped
2 cm knob of ginger, chopped
½ teaspoon shrimp paste
2 tablespoons chopped coriander roots
1 teaspoon cumin
1 shallot, trimmed and roughly chopped
3 teaspoons white peppercorns
sea salt and freshly ground black pepper,
    to taste

1   To make the red curry paste, place all the
    ingredients in a food processor or blender
    and blitz until fully combined.

2   Place a large frying pan or saucepan over
    medium heat and add the coconut oil. Add
    the shallots and curry paste and sauté for
    6–8 minutes.

3   Increase the heat to high and add the
    chicken. Stir to ensure all the chicken is
    coated in the paste mixture and cook for
    5–6 minutes.

4   Add the pumpkin and peas and stir
    through. Reduce the heat, add the coconut
    milk and simmer for a further 10–12
    minutes, stirring occasionally.

5   Remove from the heat and season with
    salt and pepper. Garnish with the chopped
    coriander leaves and serve with lime
    wedges.

Butter Chicken

This is my son's all-time favourite. Given the choice, he'd eat it every day of the week. Indian cooking ticks all the boxes for me. It's full of healthful spices and fats, and I often add some extra greenery to ensure I'm getting adequate veggies for the day.

1 tablespoon coconut oil
1 brown onion, chopped
4 garlic cloves, minced
5 cm knob of ginger, minced
1 tablespoon garam masala
1 teaspoon ground coriander
1 teaspoon curry powder
1 teaspoon turmeric
½ teaspoon cayenne pepper
1 teaspoon cumin
1 teaspoon sweet paprika
400 g chicken thigh fillets, chopped
3 tablespoons tomato purée
1 × 400 ml can coconut cream
100 g butter
sea salt and freshly ground black pepper,
    to taste
¼ bunch of coriander, chopped

1   Place a large saucepan over low heat and add the coconut oil. Add the onion, garlic and ginger and sauté for 3–4 minutes.

2   Add all the spices and stir with a wooden spoon for a further 4–5 minutes.

3   Add the chicken and stir to ensure it is coated in spices. Increase the heat to medium and cook for 5–6 minutes, or until the chicken begins to brown.

4   Stir in the tomato purée then add the coconut cream and butter. Reduce the heat to low and cook for 12–15 minutes.

5   Remove from the heat and season with salt and pepper. Sprinkle with the chopped coriander before serving.

Whole Baked Snapper with Nuoc Cham . 85

serves
4

Whole Baked Snapper
with Nuoc Cham

If you want to substitute the whole fish for fillets
in this recipe, then that's easy to do – just pan-fry
the fillets on a high heat in a little olive oil until
cooked through.

1 whole snapper, gutted and de-scaled
1 bunch of coriander
sea salt and freshly ground black pepper,
   to taste
2 lemons, halved
handful of mixed green leaves
½ punnet of medley cherry tomatoes,
   quartered
2 shallots, trimmed and chopped, to garnish

NUOC CHAM
1 small red chilli, finely chopped
1 garlic clove, finely chopped
1 tablespoon finely chopped ginger
1 tablespoon fish sauce
1 teaspoon honey
juice of 2 limes

1 Preheat your oven to 190°C. Line a baking
   tray with baking paper.

2 Pat the snapper dry using paper towel.
   Place the coriander inside the cavity of
   the fish. Place the fish on the baking tray,
   season with salt and pepper and add
   the lemon halves around it. Bake for 20
   minutes, or until the fish is cooked through
   (times vary depending on the size of the
   fish). Remove from the oven and allow to
   rest for 5 minutes.

3 To make the nuoc cham, combine all the
   ingredients in a small glass jar, cover and
   shake vigorously. Set aside.

4 In a mixing bowl, combine the green
   leaves and cherry tomatoes.

5 Sprinkle the shallots over the fish, and
   serve with the salad and nuoc cham.

serves
4

Lamb Hotpot with Carrot and Pea Smash

If you want to cook this overnight, set the oven temperature to 90°C and it'll be *so* yummy in the morning.

2 tablespoons olive oil
2 brown onions, quartered
4 garlic cloves, chopped
1 tablespoon dried rosemary
1 tablespoon dried oregano
2 bay leaves
500 g diced leg of lamb
6 whole tomatoes, cored
 and chopped
1 litre beef bone broth or stock
6 carrots, sliced
handful of button mushrooms
sea salt and freshly ground black
 pepper, to taste
1 cup peas, fresh or frozen
1 tablespoon butter

1   Preheat your oven to 250°C.

2   Place a lidded casserole or ovenproof dish over medium heat and add the olive oil. Add the onion and garlic and sauté for 3–4 minutes. Stir in the herbs and cook for a further 3 minutes.

3   Increase the heat to high and add the lamb. Cook for 4–5 minutes, or until the lamb is browned.

4   Add the tomatoes and broth and stir. Add 2 sliced carrots and the mushrooms and stir to combine. Season with salt and pepper.

5   Pop the lid on, place in the oven and reduce the temperature to 140°C. Cook for 1½ hours, or until the lamb is tender. Remove from the oven. If required, remove the lid and simmer on the stovetop to reduce the liquid.

6   Meanwhile, in a saucepan, bring some salted water to the boil and add the remaining 4 sliced carrots and the peas. Reduce the heat to a simmer and cook for 4–5 minutes. Remove from the heat and drain.

7   In a mixing bowl, combine the carrots and peas with the butter, and mash using a potato masher or fork. Season again with salt and pepper if needed.

8   Serve the mash with the lamb hotpot.

Rump Steak with Parsley and Garlic Butter

Is there a better combination than beautifully caramelised steak and garlic butter?

50 g butter
1–2 garlic cloves, minced
¼ bunch of parsley, chopped
sea salt and freshly ground black
    pepper, to taste
2 grass-fed rump steaks
2 tablespoons olive oil, plus
    1 teaspoon for cooking steak
1 teaspoon chilli flakes
1 bunch of broccolini, trimmed
juice of ½ lemon

1   In a small mixing bowl, combine the butter, garlic and parsley, or blitz in a food processor for 20 seconds. Season with salt and pepper and set aside.

2   Remove the steak from the fridge 30 minutes prior to cooking.

3   Place a large frying pan over high heat and add 1 teaspoon of olive oil. Add the steak and cook for 3 minutes on each side (for best results, flip over every 30 seconds). Once cooked to your liking, remove from the heat and allow to rest.

4   Meanwhile, place the frying pan over medium–high heat and add 2 tablespoons of olive oil with the chilli flakes. Add the broccolini and sauté for 3–5 minutes, or until they begin to soften. Remove from the heat and drizzle with lemon juice.

5   Slice the rump steak, season to taste, top with the parsley and garlic butter and broccolini, and serve.

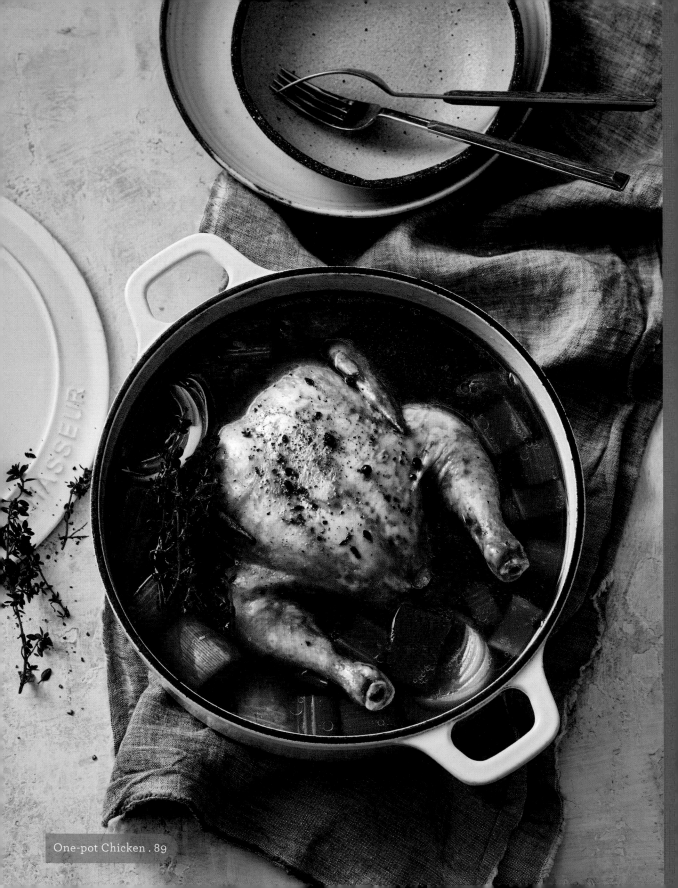

serves
4

One-pot Chicken

Bone broth is one of the most nourishing foods on the planet and should be on the radar at least weekly (if you choose to eat animal products, that is). It provides us with restorative amino acids and therapeutic properties for our gut, as well as promoting endogenous stem cells.

1 whole chicken
1 litre chicken broth or stock
2 brown onions, halved
4 garlic cloves, lightly smashed
1 leek, trimmed and chopped
4 carrots, chopped
2 bay leaves
2 celery stalks, chopped
1 sprig of thyme
1 teaspoon peppercorns
¼ bunch of parsley, roughly chopped
sea salt and freshly ground black
   pepper, to taste
1 lemon, cut into wedges, to serve

1   Place the whole chicken in a large saucepan or stockpot. Cover with broth (add more water if necessary) and bring to the boil. Reduce heat to a simmer and cook for 35 minutes; skim off any scum from the surface.

2   Add the remaining ingredients except the lemon wedges and cook for a further 30 minutes.

3   Remove from the heat and season with salt and pepper.

4   To serve, place some of the chicken meat and veggies as well as some broth into each bowl. Serve with lemon wedges.

serves
4

Crispy Fried Chook

I love cooking with chicken thigh meat. Not only is it more affordable than breast meat but it contains much more flavour. This can be a quick and easy snack for family and friends or can be added to a buffet for parties.

2 tablespoons duck fat or coconut oil
   (more if needed)
500 g chicken thigh fillets, skin on
sea salt and freshly ground black
   pepper, to taste
2 teaspoons chilli flakes
juice of ½ lemon

1   Place a large frying pan over high heat and add the fat or oil.

2   Pat the chicken dry with paper towel. Season the skin side with salt and the flesh side with the chilli flakes. Place the chicken in the hot pan, skin-side down, and cook for 6–8 minutes. Flip onto the flesh side and continue to cook for a further 3 minutes. Remove from the heat once the chicken is browned and cooked through. Allow to rest for 2–3 minutes.

3   Drizzle the lemon juice over the chicken, season with salt and pepper, and serve.

Lamb Chops with Garlic and Mint Dressing

There are few things that beat a lamb chop. The sweetness of the lamb and the delicious fat is in a world of its own.

12 grass-fed lamb chops
1 tablespoon olive oil
sea salt and freshly ground black pepper, to taste
1 lemon, cut into wedges

GARLIC AND MINT DRESSING
1 teaspoon Dijon mustard
1 tablespoon lemon juice
1 garlic clove, finely chopped
3 tablespoons olive oil
¼ bunch of mint, finely chopped

1   Take the lamb out of the fridge 30 minutes prior to cooking.

2   To make the dressing, place all the ingredients in a glass jar, cover and shake vigorously. Set aside.

3   Place a frying pan over high heat and add the olive oil. Season the chops with salt and pepper, and place in the hot pan (you may need to cook these in batches). Cook for 2–3 minutes on each side (times vary according to the thickness of the chop). Remove from the heat and allow to rest for 5 minutes.

4   Season again with salt and pepper if needed, and serve with the dressing and lemon wedges.

Pork San Choy Bau

This is an easy, delicious dish to make for the family. Kids love assembling and eating the lettuce cups.

2 tablespoons coconut oil
4 shallots, trimmed and chopped
1 red onion, chopped
4 garlic cloves, finely chopped
2 cm knob of ginger, finely chopped
2 teaspoons Chinese five-spice
2 carrots, diced
1 long red chilli, deseeded and finely chopped
120 ml chicken broth or stock
500 g pork mince
juice of 1 lime
sea salt and freshly ground black pepper, to taste
8 lettuce or Chinese cabbage cups

1   Place a large frying pan over medium heat and add the coconut oil. Add the shallots, onion, garlic and ginger and sauté for 3–4 minutes.

2   Add the five-spice, carrot and chilli and cook, stirring, for 1–2 minutes.

3   Add the chicken broth and cook for 1–2 minutes.

4   Increase the heat to high and add the pork mince. Cook for 10–12 minutes, stirring often.

5   Remove from the heat, stir in the lime juice, and season with salt and pepper. Serve with the lettuce or cabbage cups.

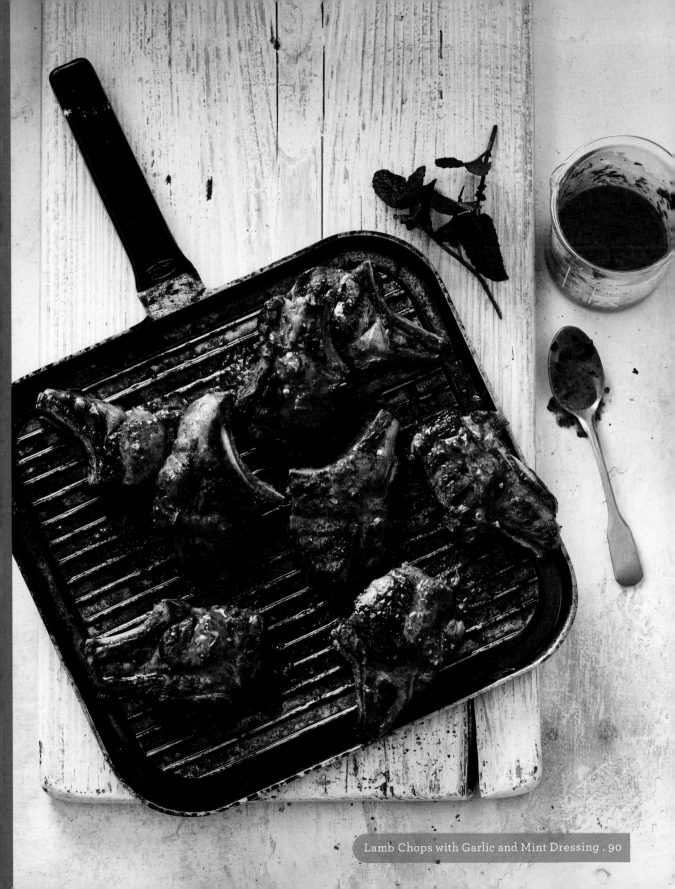

Lamb Chops with Garlic and Mint Dressing . 90

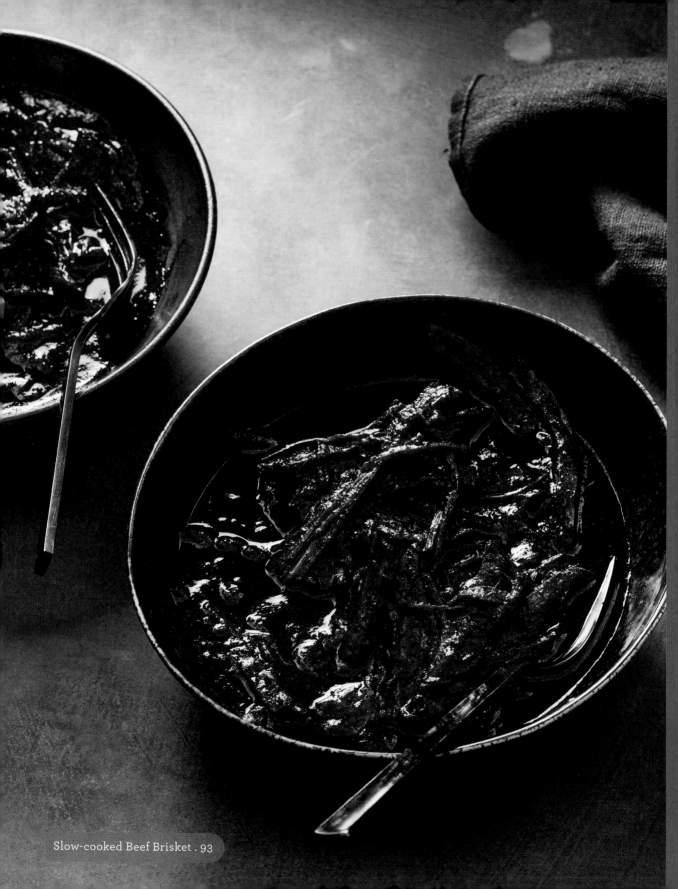

Slow-cooked Beef Brisket . 93

Slow-cooked Beef Brisket

I love a slow-cooked dish, and this one is a crowd-pleaser at any dinner party. It'll make for pretty yummy leftovers during the week at work, too ... you'll be the envy of the office.

2 tablespoons olive oil
1 onion, sliced
6 garlic cloves, chopped
1 teaspoon caraway seeds
1 teaspoon ground cumin
3 bay leaves
1 teaspoon sweet paprika
1.5 kg beef brisket, cut into quarters
250 ml red wine
600 ml tomato passata
750 ml beef bone broth or stock
sea salt and freshly ground black
    pepper, to taste

1   Preheat your oven to 250°C.

2   Place a lidded casserole or ovenproof dish over medium heat and add the olive oil. Add the onion and garlic and sauté for 3–4 minutes. Add the herbs and spices and cook for a further 1 minute.

3   Increase the heat to high and add the beef, stirring to ensure it is coated with the herbs and spices. Cook for 5–6 minutes, or until the beef is browned.

4   Add the wine and bring to the boil. Reduce the heat to a simmer and stir in the passata and broth. Season with salt and pepper.

5   Pop the lid on and place in the oven. Reduce the temperature to 160°C and cook for 4 hours, or until the beef is tender and falling apart.

6   Remove from the oven, shred the beef with two forks and return to the sauce. Season again with salt and pepper if needed, and serve.

Lamb Meatballs in Tomato Sauce

This is a favourite with the kids ... and adults, for that matter. Make them as big or as little as you want to. This recipe works equally well with beef mince.

500 g lamb mince
1 red onion, finely chopped
3 garlic cloves, finely chopped
¼ bunch of coriander, stalks and
    leaves chopped
1 teaspoon ground cumin
1 teaspoon sweet paprika
1 egg yolk
1 teaspoon Dijon mustard
sea salt and freshly ground black
    pepper, to taste
1 tablespoon butter, for frying

TOMATO SAUCE
2 tablespoons olive oil
1 red onion, chopped
2 garlic cloves, finely chopped
¼ bunch of parsley, stalks chopped,
    leaves chopped for garnish
1 × 400 g can diced tomatoes
200 ml tomato passata
sea salt and freshly ground black
    pepper, to taste

1   To make the tomato sauce: Place a large saucepan over medium heat and add the olive oil. Add the onion and garlic and sauté for 3–4 minutes. Add the parsley stalks and cook for a further 1 minute. Add the tomatoes and passata, reduce the heat to a simmer and cook for 20 minutes. Remove from the heat and season with salt and pepper.

2   Meanwhile, in a large mixing bowl, combine all the ingredients for the meatballs except the coriander leaves and butter, using your hands to ensure it is thoroughly combined. Shape the mixture into evenly sized meatballs and set aside.

3   Place a large frying pan over medium–high heat and add the butter. Add the meatballs and cook, turning often, until browned (you may have to cook them in batches).

4   Once all the meatballs are browned, place them in the tomato sauce over a low heat. Continue cooking the meatballs in the sauce until they are cooked through.

5   Remove from the heat and add the chopped coriander leaves. Season again with salt and pepper if needed, and serve.

Pork Belly with Beetroot and Apple Slaw

I remember years ago that I used to think pork belly looked amazing, but with all that fat it had to be bad for me, so I never ordered it. These days it's my first choice at cafés or restaurants. You'll love this recipe.

2 kg pork belly
2 tablespoons fennel seeds
1 teaspoon caraway seeds
1 teaspoon coriander seeds
1 teaspoon peppercorns
2 garlic cloves, skins removed
2 tablespoons coconut oil
sea salt and freshly ground black
  pepper, to taste
4 baby beetroots, grated
2 green apples, grated

1   Lightly score the skin of the pork belly diagonally in both directions. Then score the skin again, 1–2 cm deep, marking the individual portions (this makes it easier when cutting the pork belly after cooking).

2   Using a pestle and mortar, grind the fennel, caraway and coriander seeds. Add the peppercorns and grind again. Add the garlic and coconut oil and grind to make a paste.

3   Rub the paste into the pork skin, ensuring it gets into the score lines. Set aside in the fridge for a minimum of 2 hours.

4   Preheat your oven to 220°C.

5   Place the pork belly on a wire rack inside a roasting tray, season with salt and pepper and bake for 30 minutes. Then reduce the temperature to 160°C and continue to cook for 2 hours. Increase the temperature to 220°C for a further 30 minutes, or until the skin is crispy. Remove from the oven and allow to rest for 20 minutes.

6   To make the slaw, place the grated beetroot and apple in a large mixing bowl and gently toss to combine.

7   Cut the pork belly into the scored portions, and serve with the slaw.

Fried Prawns with Chilli and Salt

I still remember sitting in a restaurant in Port Douglas eating a bucket of prawns with aïoli, overlooking the ocean and watching huge gropers being fed. This recipe requires some frying, so be mindful of the hot oil.

coconut oil, for frying
3 long red chillies, deseeded and
    finely chopped
4 dozen small raw prawns
juice of 2 lemons
sea salt and freshly ground black
    pepper, to taste

1   Place a large frying pan over medium–high heat and add the coconut oil. Once hot, add the chopped chilli and the prawns (you may have to cook the prawns with chilli in batches). Cook for 1–2 minutes, or until the prawns are bright red and cooked through. Remove from the pan using a slotted spoon, allowing the oil to drain off, and transfer to a serving bowl.

2   Drizzle with lemon juice, season with salt and pepper, and serve.

Cod Tagine

This is a recipe I rustled up a few years ago – the original was delicious but so chilli-hot it was almost inedible. Don't worry, I've dialled back the chilli for this particular recipe.

1 tablespoon coconut oil
1 red onion, finely sliced
4 garlic cloves, chopped
½ stalk of lemongrass, white part only,
    finely chopped
2 cm knob of ginger, finely chopped
3–4 red chillies, deseeded and finely chopped
400 g cod (or equivalent white fish), skin
    removed, chopped
1 × 400 ml can coconut milk
100 ml water
2 zucchini, chopped
4 shallots, trimmed and chopped
1 teaspoon fish sauce
2 limes, halved
sea salt and freshly ground black pepper,
    to taste
½ bunch of coriander, chopped, for garnish

1   Preheat your oven to 150°C.

2   Place a frying pan over medium heat and add the coconut oil. Add the red onion, garlic, lemongrass, ginger and chilli and sauté for 3–4 minutes, or until they begin to soften. Remove from the heat and place into a tagine or ovenproof dish with lid.

3   Add all the remaining ingredients except the coriander to the tagine, cover and bake for 45 minutes.

4   Remove from the oven and season again with salt and pepper if needed. Add the fresh coriander before serving.

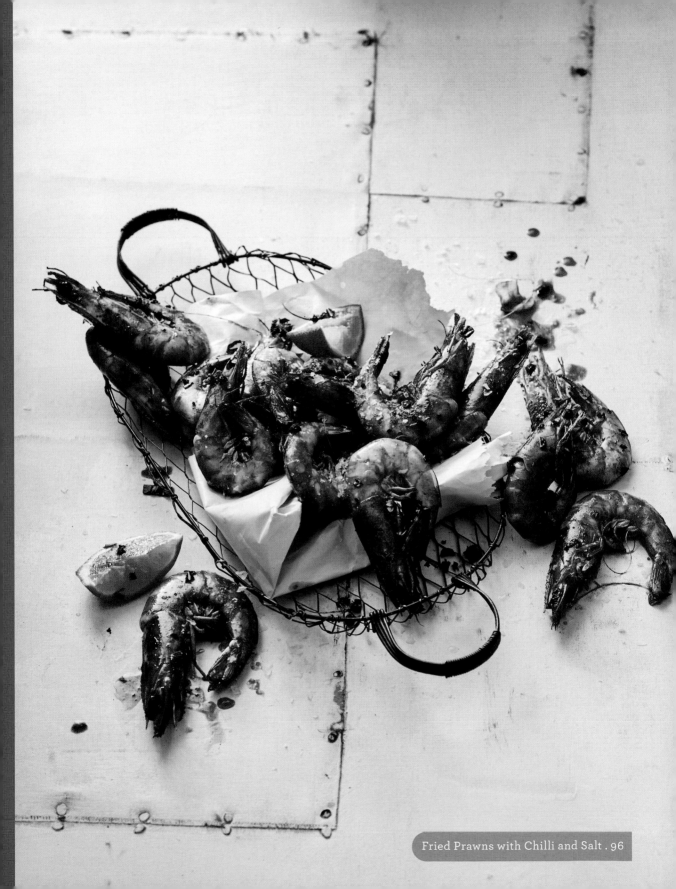

Fried Prawns with Chilli and Salt . 96

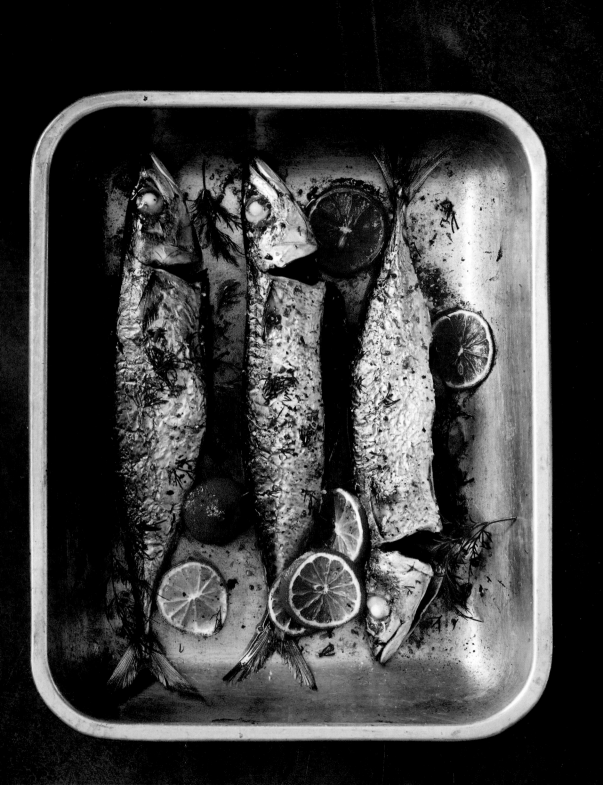

Barbecued Mackerel

When I was growing up, mackerel was often on my dinner plate and I still love the texture and flavour. My dad used to make the best Smoked Mackerel Pâté (see recipe page 129).

2 bunches of dill
4 mackerel (350 g each), gutted
2 tablespoons olive oil
sea salt and freshly ground black
    pepper, to taste
grated zest and juice of 2 lemons

1   Preheat your barbecue to high.

2   Stuff half a bunch of dill in the cavity of each fish. Drizzle the olive oil over the fish, season with salt and pepper, and sprinkle with the lemon zest.

3   Place the fish on the barbecue and cook for 3 minutes on each side. Remove from the heat and allow to rest for 2 minutes.

4   Break open the fish and drizzle with the lemon juice. Season again with salt and pepper if needed, and serve.

Crispy Broccolini with Salmon

This is a super-easy recipe that only requires a few ingredients and can be rustled up in less than ten minutes.

2 tablespoons olive oil
½ teaspoon chilli flakes
1 bunch of broccolini, trimmed
    and chopped
1 salmon portion, skin on
sea salt and freshly ground black
    pepper, to taste
juice of ½ lemon

1   Place a large frying pan over medium–high heat and add the olive oil. Add the chilli flakes and cook for 1 minute.

2   Add the broccolini, toss to coat in the olive oil and chilli, and cook for 2–3 minutes.

3   Pat the skin of the fish dry with paper towel, and season with salt and pepper. Make room in the pan for the fish by pushing the broccolini aside. Place the fish in the pan, skin-side down. Cook for 5–6 minutes on the skin side before flipping and cooking the flesh side for 2–3 minutes.

4   Remove all ingredients from the pan and allow the fish to rest for 1–2 minutes.

5   Season again with salt and pepper if needed, and drizzle with the lemon juice.

serves
4

Crispy Whitebait with Herb Mayo

Some folks find it a little confronting to eat a whole fish, but remind yourself there is additional calcium and minerals in the bones and cartilage when consuming fish like this.

coconut oil, for shallow frying
500 g whitebait, washed and drained
sea salt and freshly ground black pepper,
   to taste
juice of 1–2 lemons
2 cups Herb Mayo (see recipe page 137)

1   Place a frying pan over high heat and add the coconut oil.

2   Pat the whitebait dry with paper towel. Place the fish in the hot oil (you may need to cook these in batches). Cook for 3 minutes, or until lightly browned and crispy, before removing from the pan and allowing to drain on paper towel.

3   Season with salt and pepper, drizzle with lemon juice, and serve with the herb mayo.

serves
4

Roasted Bone Marrow with Chimichurri

Bone marrow is one of the most nutrient-dense foods on the planet, rich in omega-3 fatty acids; however, it hasn't been included here purely for nutritional benefits but for its texture and flavour. If you're looking for a delicious entrée or even a decadent snack, then this recipe is the bomb. Ask your butcher to cut up the marrow bones for you.

8–12 beef bones with marrow, cut into
   sections or lengthways
2 tablespoons olive oil
sea salt and freshly ground black pepper,
   to taste
1 cup Chimichurri (see recipe page 130)

1   Preheat your oven to 220°C.

2   Place the marrow bones on a baking tray, drizzle with olive oil and season with salt and pepper. Pop in the oven for 15 minutes, or until the bones begin to bubble.

3   Remove the bones from the oven and allow to cool for a couple of minutes. Serve with the chimichurri.

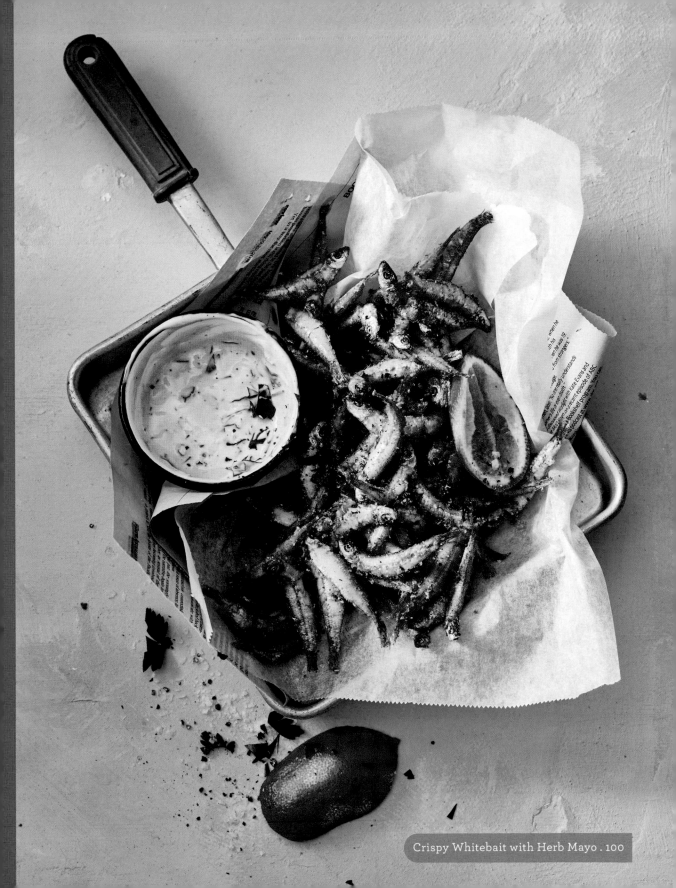

Crispy Whitebait with Herb Mayo . 100

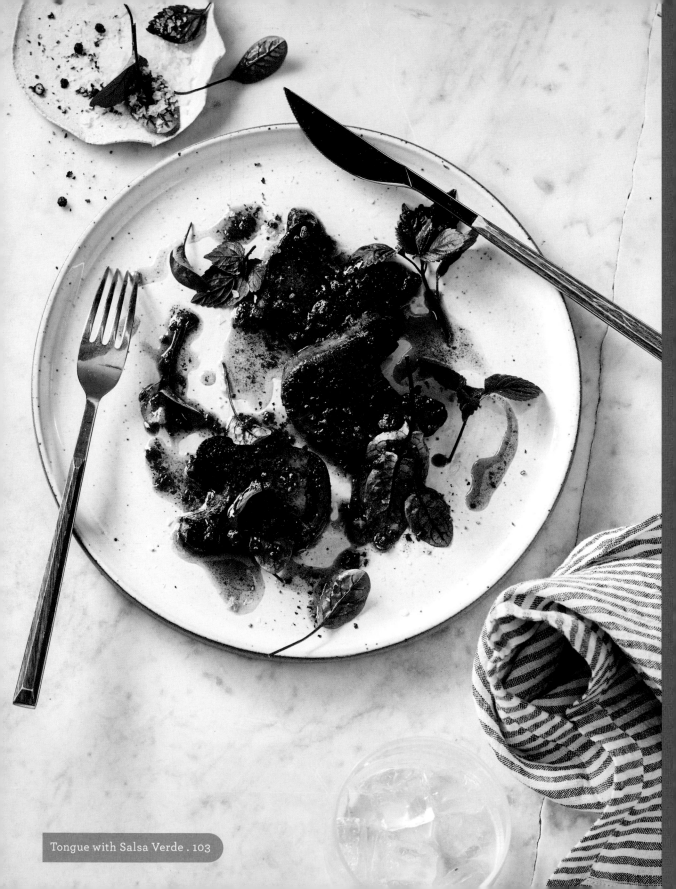

Tongue with Salsa Verde

I'm a big advocate for offal. If you choose to
eat an animal, it's important to consider the
organ meat of said animal. If you need more
persuading, organ meats are some of the most
nutrient-dense foods on the planet.

1 large ox tongue, trimmed
2 onions, quartered
1 celery stalk, chopped
1 carrot, sliced
6 peppercorns
4 garlic cloves
½ bunch of parsley, stalks included
2 bay leaves
500 ml beef bone broth or stock
   (or more if needed)
500 ml water (or more if needed)
sea salt and freshly ground black
   pepper, to taste
2 tablespoons olive oil
1 cup Salsa Verde (see recipe page 133)

1   Soak the tongue in salted cold water for
    1 hour. Rinse under cold running water
    and place the tongue in a large saucepan.

2   Add all the other ingredients except the
    olive oil and salsa verde (add more liquid
    if necessary – the tongue needs to be
    submerged). Bring to the boil over high
    heat then reduce heat to a simmer and
    cook for 1½ hours, or until the tongue is
    cooked through (a skewer should go in
    easily). Remove from the pan and allow to
    cool. Once cooled, peel the skin off to reveal
    the meat, and slice into 1–1½ cm discs.

3   Place a frying pan over high heat and add
    the olive oil. Add the sliced tongue and
    cook for 1 minute on each side, or until you
    get some caramelisation.

4   Remove from the heat and serve with
    salsa verde.

serves
4

Beef Bolognese
with Liver and
Zucchini Ribbons

This recipe works exceptionally well without the liver, but if you're new to cooking or eating offal then it's a great entry-level option. The liver (you can also substitute with kidney) is enough to amplify the nutrient density but equally won't change the flavour dramatically.

3 tablespoons olive oil
2 small brown onions, finely chopped
4 garlic cloves, finely chopped
1 celery stalk, finely chopped
1 tablespoon oregano
1 tablespoon dried basil
1 tablespoon dried thyme
2 bay leaves
500 g beef mince
100 g lamb's liver, trimmed and chopped
500 ml beef bone broth or stock
2 × 400 g cans diced tomatoes
300 ml tomato passata
2 carrots, grated
6 button mushrooms, quartered
sea salt and freshly ground black
    pepper, to taste
2 zucchini, cut into ribbons

1   Place a large saucepan or frying pan over medium heat and add the olive oil. Add the onion, garlic and celery and sauté for 3–4 minutes. Add the dried herbs and cook for a further 1–2 minutes.

2   Add the mince and liver, increase the heat to high and cook until browned.

3   Reduce the heat to medium, add the broth and cook for 5–6 minutes.

4   Add the tomatoes and passata, stir and cook for 3–4 minutes.

5   Add the carrot and mushrooms and cook for a further 5–6 minutes. Remove from the heat and season with salt and pepper.

6   Before serving, add the zucchini ribbons to the mince and toss through.

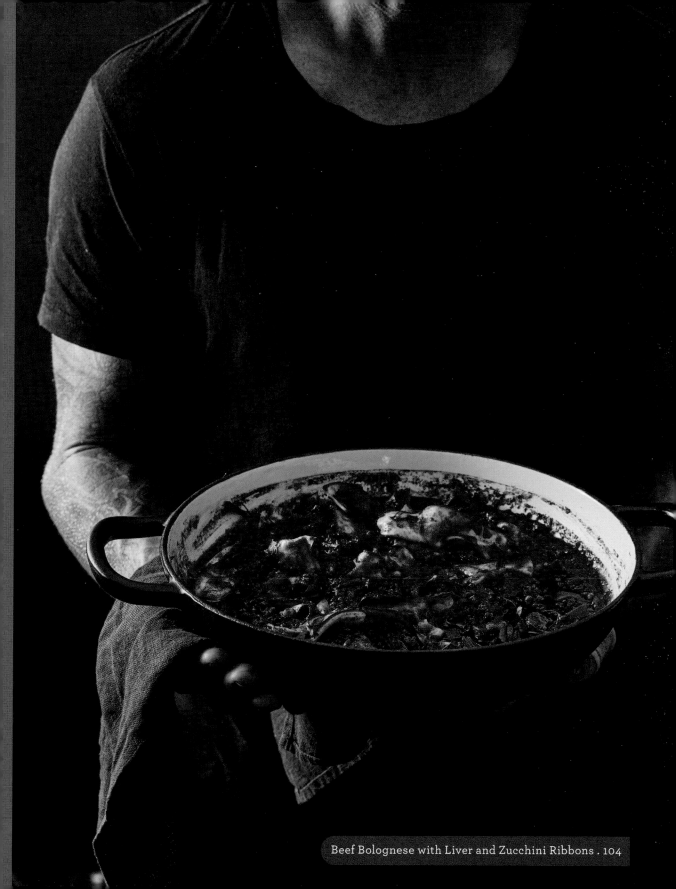

Beef Bolognese with Liver and Zucchini Ribbons . 104

Fried Chicken Liver
with Chimichurri

This recipe is pretty simple and works well
served with lettuce cups.

1 tablespoon olive oil
3 eschalots, halved
½ bunch of parsley, stalks chopped
    and leaves picked
4 garlic cloves, halved
1 tablespoon baby capers, rinsed
    and drained
500 g chicken livers, trimmed
juice of 1 lemon
sea salt and freshly ground black
    pepper, to taste
½ cup Chimichurri (see recipe page 130)

1   Place a frying pan over medium heat and
    add the olive oil. Add the eschalots, parsley
    stalks and garlic and sauté for 3–4 minutes.

2   Add the baby capers and cook for a further
    1 minute.

3   Increase the heat to high, add the chicken
    livers and cook for 4–5 minutes, or until
    browned and cooked (a little pink on the
    inside is fine). Remove from the heat and
    allow to rest for 1 minute.

4   Drizzle with lemon juice, season with salt
    and pepper, sprinkle with parsley leaves
    and serve with the chimichurri.

Fried Chicken Liver with Chimichurri . 106

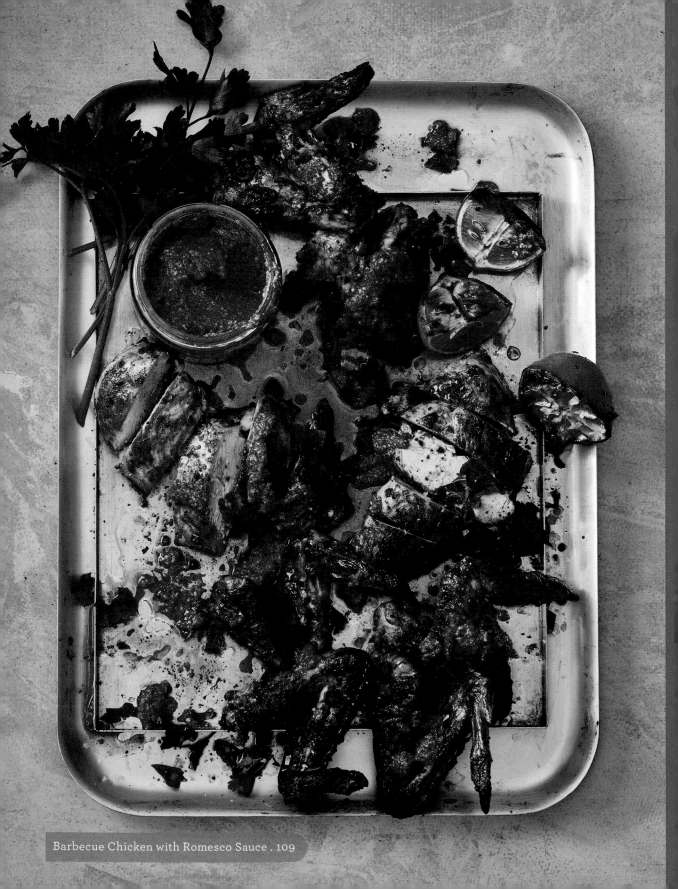

Barbecue Chicken with Romesco Sauce . 109

Barbecue Chicken with Romesco Sauce

This is so tasty; it'll be a crowd-pleaser at your next barbecue and a recipe you'll be cooking for many more summers to come.

2 chicken breast fillets
2 tablespoons olive oil
sea salt and freshly ground black
　pepper, to taste
juice of 1 lemon
¼ bunch of parsley, chopped
4 tablespoons Romesco Sauce
　(see recipe page 134)

1　Remove the chicken from the fridge at least 30 minutes prior to cooking.

2　Preheat your barbecue to high.

3　Coat the chicken with olive oil and season with salt and pepper. Place on the barbecue and cook for 12–15 minutes (depending on size), turning halfway through cooking. Remove from the heat, cover with foil and allow to rest for 5 minutes.

4　Slice the chicken breast across the grain, drizzle with lemon juice and season again with salt and pepper if needed. Sprinkle with chopped parsley and serve with the Romesco Sauce.

Lamb Bolognese with Zucchini Ribbons

3 tablespoons olive oil
2 small brown onions, finely chopped
4 garlic cloves, finely chopped
1 celery stalk, finely chopped
1 tablespoon dried basil
1 tablespoon dried thyme
2 bay leaves
500 g lamb mince
500 ml beef bone broth or stock
2 × 400 g cans diced tomatoes
300 ml tomato passata
1 carrot, grated
6 button mushrooms, quartered
sea salt and freshly ground black
　pepper, to taste
2 zucchini, cut into ribbons

1　Place a large saucepan or frying pan over medium heat and add the olive oil. Add the onion, garlic and celery and sauté for 3–4 minutes. Add the dried herbs and cook for a further 1–2 minutes.

2　Add the lamb mince, increase the heat to high and cook until browned.

3　Reduce the heat to medium, add the broth and cook for 5–6 minutes. Add the tomatoes and passata, stir and cook for 3–4 minutes.

4　Add the carrot and mushrooms and cook for a further 5–6 minutes. Remove from the heat and season with salt and pepper.

5　Before serving, add the zucchini ribbons to the mince and toss through.

serves
2

Raphie's Okra and Bean Curry

This vegetarian curry can be a side dish or a stand-alone curry, and the taste is unreal. Thanks for sharing, Raphie!

3 tablespoons ghee
¾ teaspoon mustard seeds
1 onion, sliced
4 garlic cloves, minced
2 cm knob of ginger, minced
1 long green chilli, chopped
¾ teaspoon fennel seeds
1 teaspoon turmeric
½ teaspoon ground cumin
2 cinnamon sticks
10 fresh curry leaves
150 g okra, halved lengthways
150 g green beans, trimmed
1 × 400 ml can coconut cream
sea salt and freshly ground black
   pepper, to taste

1   Place a saucepan over medium heat and add the ghee. Add the mustard seeds and cook, stirring, for 2–3 minutes.

2   Add the onion, garlic, ginger, chilli, fennel seeds, spices and curry leaves, and cook for 1–2 minutes. Add the okra and beans, stir to ensure they are coated in the spices, and cook for a further 2–3 minutes.

3   Add the coconut cream, reduce the heat to low and simmer until the vegetables have softened. Remove from the heat, season with salt and pepper, and serve.

serves
4

Pork Chops with Celeriac and Carrot Mash

You don't have to go without mash if you select some lower-carb veggies and add plenty of delicious fat. Even white potato can feature in a keto diet, dependent on volume and the level of resistant starch. It's actually possible to reduce the carb value of white potato – see *The Keto Diet* for more details.

4 carrots, chopped
1 celeriac, chopped
3 tablespoons butter
   (or more if needed)
4 pork chops
2 tablespoons coconut cream
sea salt and freshly ground black
   pepper, to taste

1   Bring a pot of salted water to the boil. Place the carrots and celeriac into the water, return to the boil then reduce heat to a simmer.

2   Meanwhile, place a frying pan over high heat and add 1 tablespoon of the butter. Add the pork chops and cook for 3–4 minutes on each side, until browned and cooked through. Remove from the heat and allow to rest.

3   Once the vegetables are softened, remove from the heat and drain. Add the remaining butter and the coconut cream, and mash using a masher. Season the mash with salt and pepper, and add more butter if needed.

4   Serve the pork chops with the mash.

Raphie's Okra and Bean Curry . 110

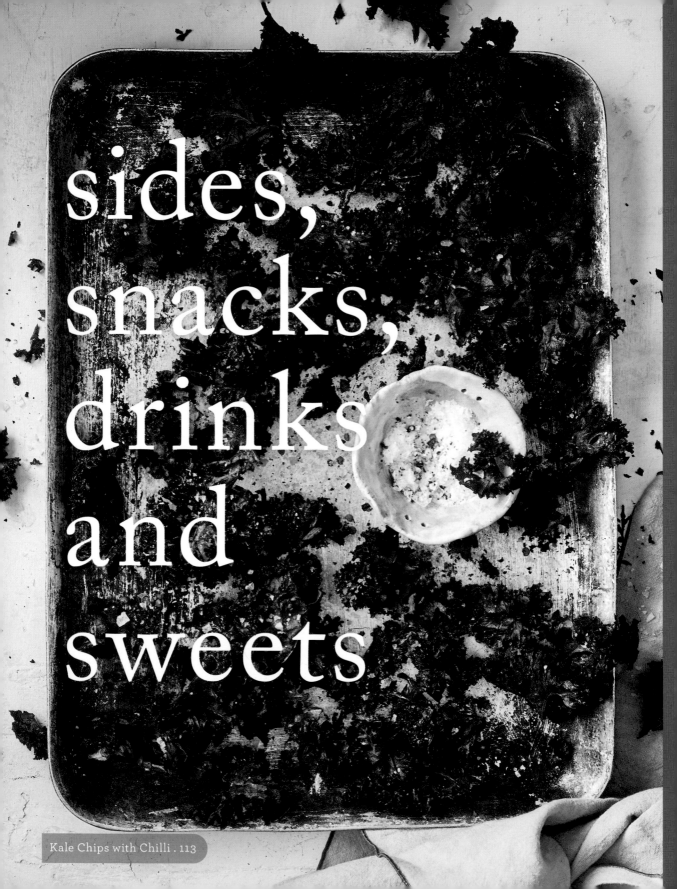

sides, snacks, drinks and sweets

serves
2

serves
2

Kale Chips with Chilli

After burning several batches of these on a cooking show, I vowed never to make them again as long as I live. A recent show with Dr Terry Wahls reignited my love for them. This is such an easy recipe, and it's very possible not to burn them!

½ bunch of kale, stems removed and
    leaves torn
1 tablespoon coconut oil
1 teaspoon sweet paprika
1 teaspoon chilli flakes
sea salt and freshly ground black pepper,
    to taste

1   Preheat your oven to 180°C and line a baking tray with baking paper.

2   In a large mixing bowl, combine the kale leaves and coconut oil. Massage the oil into the leaves using your hands. Add the paprika and chilli flakes and stir to combine. Season with salt and pepper.

3   Transfer to the baking tray and bake for 25 minutes, gently tossing halfway through baking. Remove from the oven when the chips have browned slightly on the edges. Allow the chips to cool and crisp up.

4   Season again with salt and pepper, and serve.

Simple Kale Salad

Surprisingly, this is one of my son's favourite salads – kale isn't everybody's cup of tea but this is a winner with him. There are many different ways to treat kale, so if you don't love it raw, try it baked or sautéed.

½ bunch of kale, trimmed and finely chopped
1 punnet of cherry tomatoes, halved
¼ cup pepitas

DRESSING
1 tablespoon apple cider vinegar
3 tablespoons olive oil
1 teaspoon Dijon mustard
juice of ½ lemon
sea salt and freshly ground black pepper,
    to taste

1   To make the dressing, combine all the ingredients in a small jar, cover and shake vigorously. Set aside.

2   In a large mixing bowl, combine the kale, tomatoes and pepitas, and gently toss together.

3   Add the dressing and gently toss through. Season again with salt and pepper if needed, and serve.

serves
2

Slow-cooked Tomatoes with Spinach

This rustic dish also makes for a delicious lunch. The key is not to rush the garlic – allow it to sit in the fat and cook for a while on a low heat, then, as it begins to soften, add the other ingredients. The fat will take on the nuttiness and sweetness of the garlic.

2 tablespoons olive oil
2 tablespoons ghee
6 garlic cloves, lightly crushed
2 punnets of cherry tomatoes, halved
1 bunch of English spinach, roughly chopped
juice of 1 lemon
sea salt and freshly ground black pepper,
   to taste

1   Place a saucepan over low heat and add the olive oil and ghee. Add the garlic and cook for 6 minutes, stirring occasionally.

2   Add the tomatoes and pop the lid on. Cook for a further 6 minutes.

3   Remove the lid, add the chopped spinach and cook, stirring, for 1–2 minutes.

4   Remove from the heat, toss with the lemon juice, and season with salt and pepper.

serves
4

Brussels with Bacon

1 tablespoon tallow or lard
150 g bacon, diced
400 g Brussels sprouts, trimmed and halved
1 teaspoon sweet paprika
sea salt and freshly ground black pepper,
   to taste
juice of 1 lemon

1   Place a large frying pan over medium-high heat and add the tallow or lard. Add the bacon and cook, stirring often, for 5–6 minutes, or until the bacon fat has rendered and crispy bits have formed. Remove the bacon and set aside, but leave some bacon fat in the pan.

2   Add the Brussels sprouts and paprika and toss to combine. Cook, tossing occasionally, until the sprouts have almost crisped on the outside and are slightly soft on the inside. Add the bacon and stir for 1 minute.

3   Remove from the heat and season with salt and pepper. Toss with lemon juice and serve.

Buttery Mixed Mushrooms

I've been making a version of this since I was old enough to navigate around the kitchen – getting in the way of the chefs in my family's pub. There's something very alluring about the combination of butter, mushrooms and lemon.

2 tablespoons butter (or more if needed)
1 tablespoon olive oil (or more if needed)
300 g mixed mushrooms (brown, Swiss, shiitake, enoki), roughly chopped
2 sprigs of thyme
juice of 1 lemon
sea salt and freshly ground black pepper, to taste

1   Place a large frying pan over low-medium heat and add the butter and olive oil. Add the mushrooms and thyme and gently toss. Cook for 8–10 minutes, or until the mushrooms have softened. Add more butter or olive oil if necessary, as the mushrooms will absorb a great deal.

2   Remove from the heat, toss with the lemon juice, and season with salt and pepper.

Asparagus with Herb Butter

Since I was a little kid, I've loved the texture and flavour of asparagus. It was always something I'd order when my folks took my sis and me to our favourite restaurant. The trick then, as it is now, is to complement the asparagus with butter and black pepper.

40 asparagus spears
2–3 tablespoons herb butter or Café de Paris Butter (see recipe page 137)
sea salt and freshly ground black pepper, to taste

1   Bring a large pot of salted water to the boil.

2   Trim the asparagus (ensure you don't discard all of the stem, only the very end).

3   Once the water is boiling, add the asparagus and cook for 90 seconds. Remove from the water and drain.

4   Place in a bowl, add the butter and toss to coat the asparagus. Season with salt and pepper, and serve.

Whole Baked Cauliflower

This is a real crowd-pleaser and looks great on the table as a centrepiece. Once you've tried this, you'll never go back to thinking veggies are boring.

½ cup coconut oil
1 teaspoon fennel seeds
1 teaspoon coriander seeds
1 teaspoon cumin seeds
1 tablespoon garam masala
1 head of cauliflower, stalk and leaves
  trimmed
sea salt and freshly ground black
  pepper, to taste
juice of 1 lemon

1   Preheat your oven to 190°C.

2   Place a frying pan over medium heat and add the coconut oil. Add the seeds and garam masala and cook, stirring, for 2–3 minutes, or until the spices become fragrant. Remove from the heat.

3   Place the cauliflower in a baking tray. Baste all over with the oil and spice mix, and season with salt and pepper. Bake for 30 minutes then remove from the oven and baste again. Pop back into the oven and bake for a further 30 minutes, or until the stem is tender.

4   Remove from the oven, season again with salt and pepper, drizzle over the lemon juice, and serve.

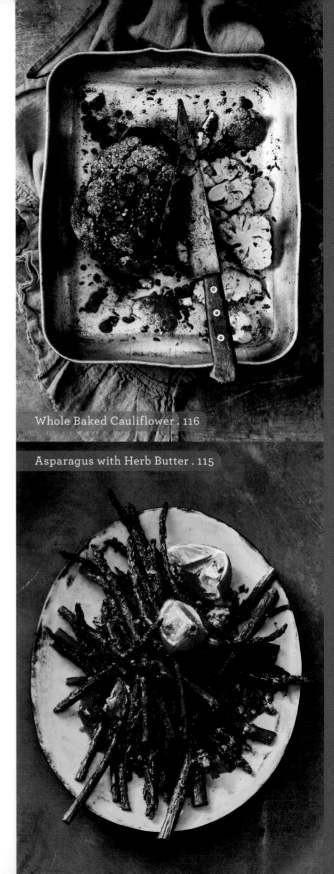

Whole Baked Cauliflower . 116

Asparagus with Herb Butter . 115

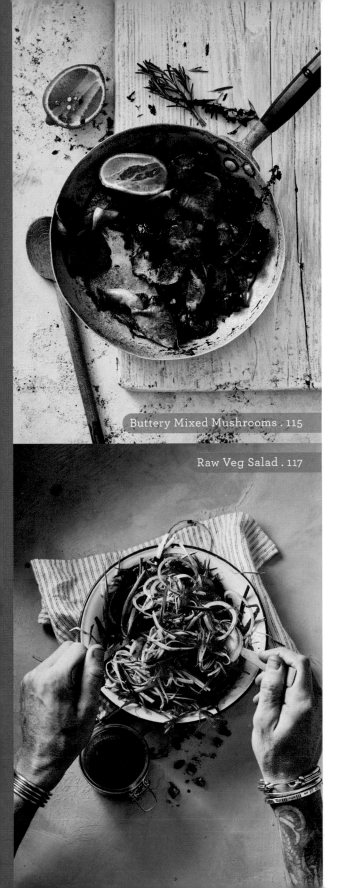

Buttery Mixed Mushrooms . 115

Raw Veg Salad . 117

serves
2

Raw Veg Salad

If you don't feel immediately healthier after eating this salad, it's maybe time to throw in the towel, haha! I'm a great advocate for making veggies the hero of our plate, and this is a recipe that certainly helps to do that.

3 carrots, grated
3 small zucchini, grated
2 medium beetroot, grated
1 red onion, thinly sliced
1 red capsicum, julienned
½ cup raw walnuts
¼ cup pepitas

DRESSING
5–6 tablespoons olive oil
2 tablespoons apple cider vinegar
2 long red chillies, finely chopped
¼ bunch of coriander, chopped
sea salt and freshly ground black
    pepper, to taste

1   To make the dressing, combine all the ingredients in a glass jar, cover and shake vigorously. Set aside.

2   Place all the ingredients for the salad in a large mixing bowl and lightly toss to combine.

3   Add the dressing and toss through, season again with salt and pepper if needed, and serve.

serves
4

Baked Pumpkin with Tahini Dressing

There's something incredibly warming and comforting about baked pumpkin, and this version won't disappoint in that department. Serve this with some baked fish or lamb and the day is made.

½ jap pumpkin, skin on, cut into wedges
2 tablespoons olive oil
2 teaspoons ground cumin
1 teaspoon cinnamon
sea salt and freshly ground black
   pepper, to taste
juice of 1 lime
3 tablespoons Tahini Dressing
   (see recipe page 131)
¼ bunch of coriander, chopped

1   Preheat your oven to 220°C and line a baking tray with baking paper.

2   In a large mixing bowl, combine the pumpkin, olive oil and spices. Lightly toss to ensure all the pumpkin is coated in oil and spice.

3   Place the pumpkin skin-side down on the baking tray. Season with salt and pepper. Bake for 25 minutes, or until browned and cooked through.

4   Remove from the oven, transfer to a serving plate and drizzle with the lime juice and tahini dressing. Sprinkle with coriander, season again with salt and pepper, and serve.

serves
12

Sauerkraut

Once reserved only for breakfast on European holidays, sauerkraut and fermented food generally have made a resurgence in the health-food community. The live cultures in fermented foods are what you want to help foster a healthy and happy gut.

1 litre still mineral water
40 g fine sea salt and freshly ground
   black pepper
½ red cabbage, trimmed and core removed,
   chopped into 5 mm-wide strips
150 g carrot, coarsely grated
3 bay leaves

1   Combine the water and salt, stir until a brine is made, and set aside.

2   In a large mixing bowl, combine the cabbage, carrot and bay leaves.

3   Place the vegetables in a clean 2-litre preserving jar. Using the end of a clean rolling pin, press them down to compact. Leave some room at the top of the jar, about 5 cm.

4   Pour the brine into the jar. The vegetables need to remain submerged, so use some pickling weights to ensure they stay weighed down under the brine.

5   Close the lid and place the jar on a plate to catch any seepage. Store in a cool room for 7 days.

6   Test the cabbage for sourness and tang; if it's not quite there in taste, reseal the jar (replace the weights, too) and store for a further 3–4 days.

Baked Pumpkin with Tahini Dressing . 118

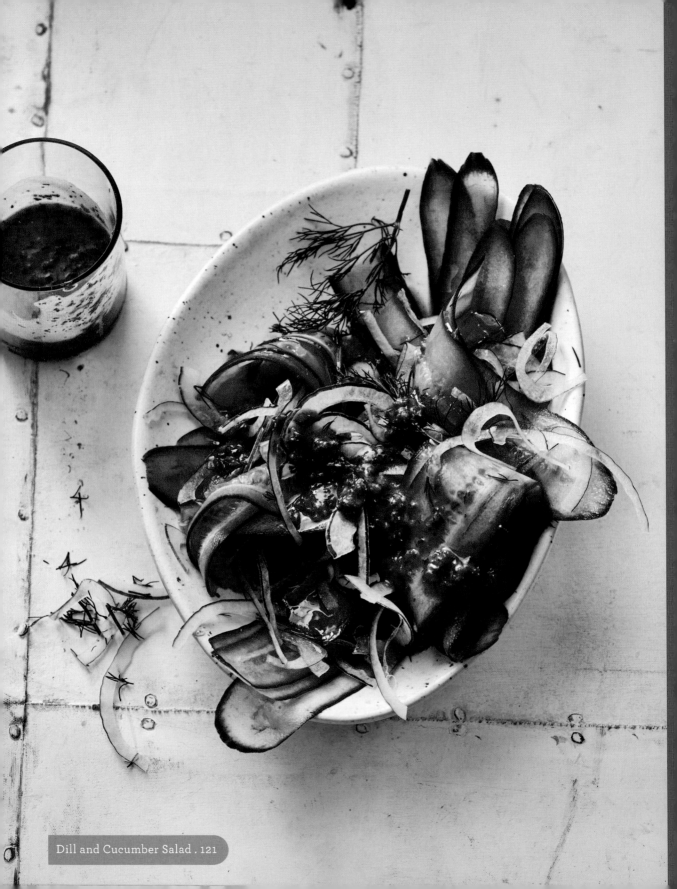

Dill and Cucumber Salad

Simple and fuss-free, this incredibly light dish is a perfect salad to make to accompany a fatty piece of fish.

2 cucumbers, halved and thinly sliced
½ bunch of dill, chopped
1 red onion, thinly sliced

DRESSING
1 teaspoon Dijon mustard
2 tablespoons apple cider vinegar
juice of ½ lemon
5 tablespoons olive oil
¼ bunch of parsley, chopped
¼ bunch of dill, chopped
sea salt and freshly ground black
  pepper, to taste

1 To make the dressing, combine all the ingredients in a glass jar, cover and shake vigorously. Set aside.

2 In a large mixing bowl, combine the cucumber, dill and red onion.

3 Add 2–3 tablespoons of the dressing and lightly toss until evenly distributed. Season with salt and pepper, and serve.

Macadamia Pesto

1 bunch of basil, leaves picked
¼ bunch of mint, leaves picked
½ garlic clove
½ cup raw macadamias
¼ cup olive oil or avocado oil
  (or more if needed)
juice of ½ lemon
sea salt and freshly ground black
  pepper, to taste

1 Throw all the ingredients in a blender or food processor. Blitz for 20–30 seconds, or until fully combined. Add more oil if required.

Matilda's Zero-effort Nibble

If I didn't include a recipe from the girlfriend in this book, I'd never hear the last of it. Matilda has chosen to share a super-quick and easy snack. It literally takes two minutes to make.

1 Lebanese cucumber, sliced
1 red capsicum, sliced
1 celery stalk, sliced
1 tablespoon tahini
1 avocado, diced
juice of 1 lemon
sea salt and freshly ground black
 pepper, to taste

1 Throw all the ingredients in a bowl and lightly toss to combine.

2 Transfer to a plate, season again with salt and pepper if needed, and serve.

Grain-free Bread

With bread being a staple for so many people, here's a terrific grain-free version.

1 tablespoon butter
2 cups almond meal
1 cup arrowroot
2 tablespoons chia seeds
1 teaspoon bicarbonate of soda
4 tablespoons pepitas
1 teaspoon sea salt
6 eggs
2 teaspoons apple cider vinegar
2 cups grated zucchini
1 carrot, grated
sea salt, extra, and freshly ground black
 pepper

1 Preheat your oven to 160°C. Grease a loaf tin with the butter.

2 In a bowl, combine the almond meal, arrowroot, chia seeds, bicarb soda, 2 tablespoons of the pepitas and the salt.

3 In a separate bowl, combine the eggs, apple cider vinegar, zucchini and carrot.

4 Combine both the wet and dry ingredients until a dough is formed.

5 Place the dough into the loaf tin and sprinkle the remaining pepitas on top. Season with salt and pepper. Bake for 1 hour, or until golden and cooked through.

6 Remove from the oven and allow to cool on a wire rack.

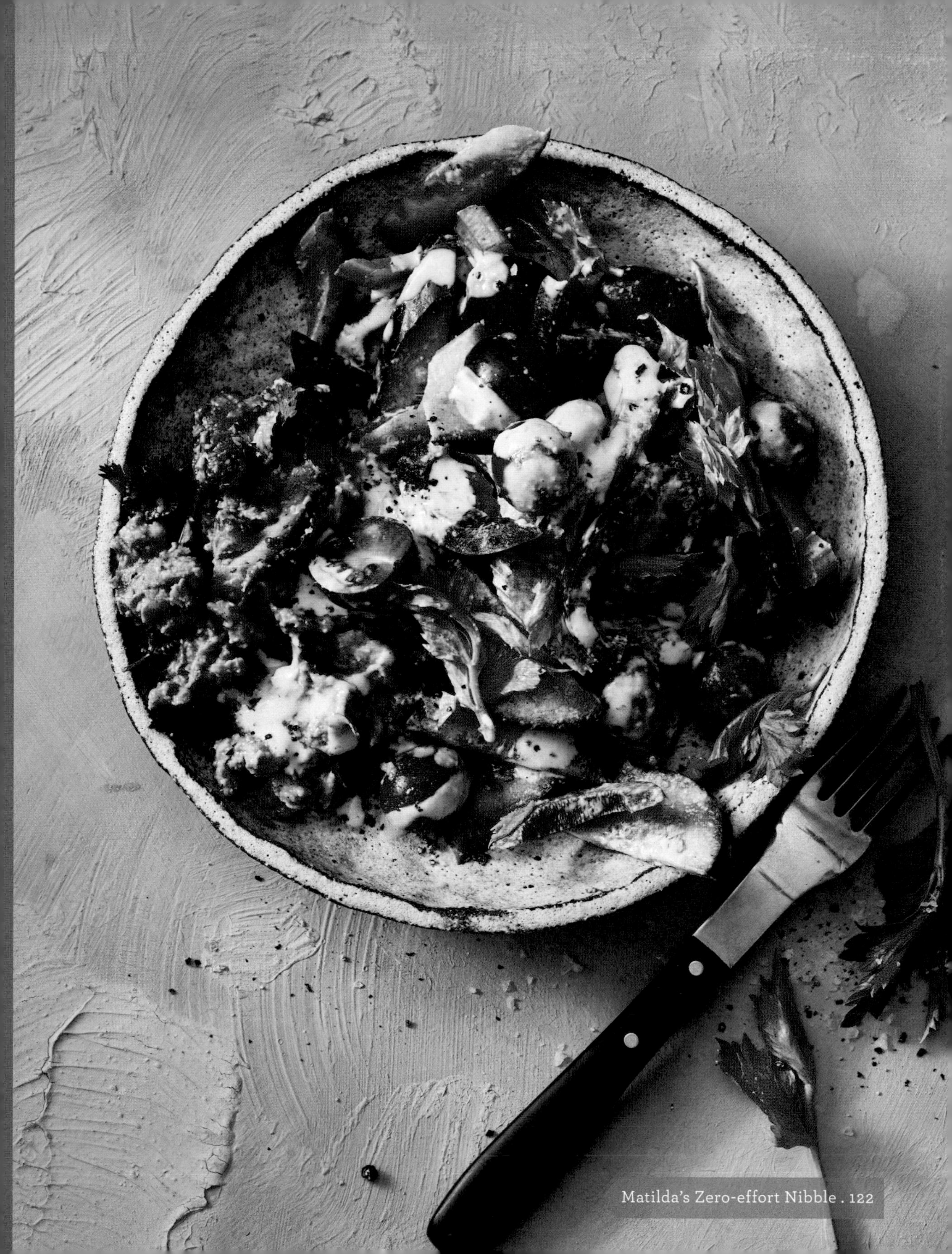

Matilda's Zero-effort Nibble . 122

Honorine's Coconut Sambal

This recipe comes courtesy of Honorine Misso, a passionate home-cook whose love and knowledge of Sri Lankan cuisine is unsurpassed. You're going to absolutely love this dish. It'll go well with a curry.

1 cup desiccated coconut
60 ml water
½ onion, diced
¼ teaspoon chilli flakes
3 teaspoons Kashmiri chilli powder (not hot)
1 tablespoon lime juice
sea salt and freshly ground black pepper,
    to taste

1   In a large bowl, combine the coconut and water. Add the remaining ingredients and combine using your hands.

2   Transfer to an airtight container and refrigerate.

Baba Ganoush

2 large eggplants
2 garlic cloves
juice of ½ lemon (or more if needed)
3 teaspoons olive oil (or more if needed)
2 tablespoons tahini
1 teaspoon ground cumin
sea salt and freshly ground black pepper,
    to taste

1   Preheat your oven to 200°C.

2   Pierce several holes in the skin of the eggplants. Place on a baking tray and bake for 40 minutes, or until the insides have softened. Remove from the oven and allow to cool.

3   Cut the eggplants in half lengthways, scoop out the flesh and place in a blender or food processor. Add the remaining ingredients and blitz for 20–30 seconds, or until fully combined. Add more lemon juice or olive oil according to taste.

makes
1
batch

Anchovy Dip

Anchovies aren't everybody's favourite fish – perhaps it's because of their 'hairy' texture, or the notion of eating a fillet with bones – but hopefully this dip will convince anyone sitting on the anchovy fence.

300 ml unsweetened coconut yoghurt
6–8 anchovy fillets
1 tablespoon lemon juice
½ teaspoon dried rosemary
sea salt and freshly ground black pepper, to taste

1   In a large mixing bowl, combine all the ingredients together, mashing the anchovies. Season with salt and pepper.

serves
6

Seed Crackers

Don't be put off by the cooking time for these crackers – they are well worth the wait!

150 g linseeds
100 g mixed seeds (sunflower seeds, sesame seeds, pepitas)
1 teaspoon ground cumin
½ teaspoon sweet paprika
sea salt and freshly ground black pepper, to taste

1   Place the linseeds in one bowl and the mixed seeds in another and add enough water to both to cover. Set aside to soak overnight.

2   Drain both batches of seeds, then place in a bowl and combine. Add the spices and season with salt and pepper.

3   Transfer to a blender and blitz (pulse) until slightly processed but with some whole seeds.

4   Preheat your oven to 50°C and line two baking trays with baking paper.

5   Spread and press a thin layer of seeds evenly on each tray. Bake for 6 hours (turning over at the 3-hour mark).

6   Remove from the oven and allow to cool on wire racks.

7   Cut the seed crackers and serve with a pâté or dip of your choice.

serves
4

Chicken Liver Pâté

This recipe is so quick and easy and provides you with one of the most nutrient-rich dishes around. Liver and various other forms of offal are the royalty of health foods, up there with seaweed and some spices for nutrient density.

1 tablespoon butter
1 brown onion, chopped
2 garlic cloves, chopped
2 sprigs of rosemary
2 sprigs of thyme
400 g chicken livers, trimmed and chopped
250 ml chicken broth or stock
50 g butter
sea salt and freshly ground black pepper,
  to taste
¼ cup melted coconut oil, for topping the pâté

1   Place a frying pan over medium heat and add the butter. Add the onion, garlic and herbs and sauté for 3–4 minutes.

2   Add the chicken livers and cook for 5–6 minutes, until browned.

3   Add the broth, reduce the heat and simmer for a further 8–10 minutes.

4   Remove from the heat, discard the sprigs of herbs and transfer to a blender or food processor.

5   Add the butter, season with salt and pepper, and blitz until creamy and smooth. Remove from the jug and transfer to a ramekin, smoothing the top using a spoon or palate knife.

6   Allow the pâté to cool before pouring on the coconut oil to act as a seal. Pop in the fridge.

theketodietcookbook

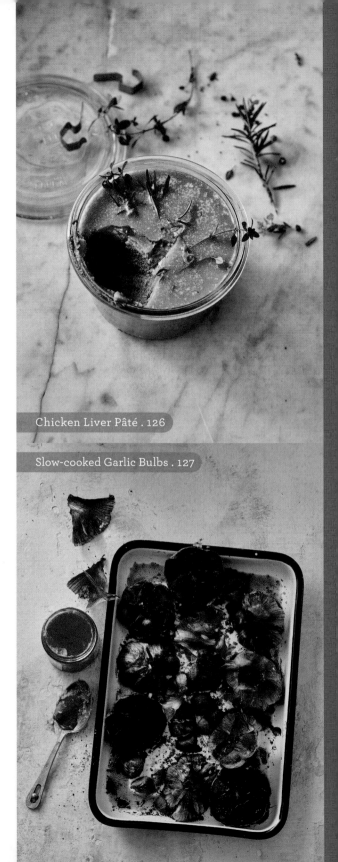

Chicken Liver Pâté . 126

Slow-cooked Garlic Bulbs . 127

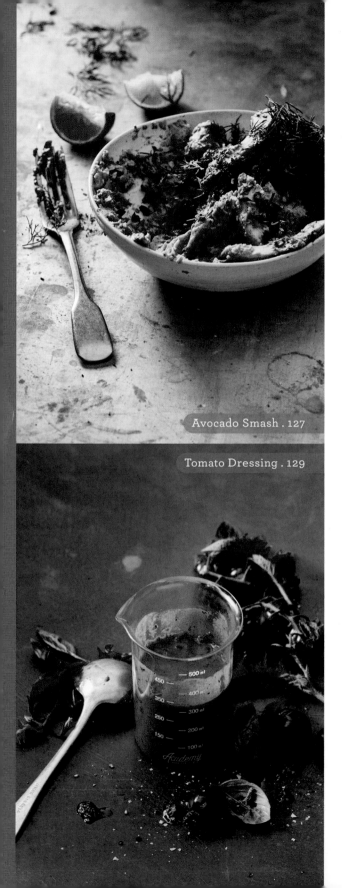

Avocado Smash . 127

Tomato Dressing . 129

Slow-cooked Garlic Bulbs

Slow-roasted garlic makes me weak at the knees.
Add a bulb or three to any tray of roasted veg.

12 garlic bulbs, cut in half
3 tablespoons olive oil
¼ cup ghee

1   Preheat your oven to 160°C and line a
    baking tray with baking paper.

2   Place the bulbs cut-side down on the tray.
    Drizzle with the olive oil and bake for
    45 minutes, or until browned and cooked
    through.

3   Store in an airtight container in the fridge.

serves
2

Avocado Smash

This can be eaten as a snack or combined with
fish or salad to add some fat to the dish.

2 ripe avocados, flesh scooped out
¼ bunch of dill, roughly chopped
½ teaspoon chilli flakes
juice of 1 lime
1 teaspoon olive oil
sea salt and freshly ground black pepper,
    to taste

1   In a large mixing bowl, gently mash the
    avocado with a fork.

2   Add the remaining ingredients and gently
    fork through until combined.

Macadamia 'Cheese'

Let's celebrate our little native nut, as it's one of the most healthful nuts on the planet with its omega 3:6 ratio. Also check out my Triple Nut Choc Spread recipe on page 138.

2 cups raw macadamias, soaked in water
    for a minimum of 6 hours
juice of 1 lemon
1 cup water
sea salt and freshly ground black pepper,
    to taste

1   Drain the macadamias and place in a blender or food processor. Add the lemon juice and blitz for 20–30 seconds. Gradually add the water until the 'cheese' reaches the desired consistency.

2   Season with salt and pepper, and store in an airtight container in the fridge.

Tapenade

1 cup kalamata olives, pitted
1 garlic clove
4 anchovy fillets
1 tablespoon baby capers
¼ cup olive oil

1   Throw all the ingredients in a blender or food processor. Blitz for 20–30 seconds, or until fully combined. Store in the fridge.

Mango and Lime Dressing

This is a delicious dressing that marries well with salad or fish. Try it with grilled sardines.

1 mango, flesh removed
grated zest and juice of 1 lime
1 teaspoon Dijon mustard
1 teaspoon rice wine vinegar
2 tablespoons olive oil
sea salt and freshly ground black pepper,
    to taste

1   Place all the ingredients in a glass jar, cover and shake vigorously. Store in the fridge.

Smoked Mackerel Pâté

My dad was a bit of a whizz in the kitchen, always trying new flavour combinations and dishes. Not all of his experiments worked 100 per cent of the time – that's the price of being experimental – but his pâtés were always spot-on.

2 whole smoked mackerel, skin and bones removed
1 teaspoon freshly grated horseradish
2 teaspoons Dijon mustard
2 tablespoons coconut yoghurt or cream
juice of ½ lemon (more to taste if needed)
100 g unsalted butter
sea salt and freshly ground black pepper, to taste

1   Throw all the ingredients in a blender or food processor and blitz for 20 seconds, or until smooth.

2   Season again with salt and pepper if needed, then transfer to an airtight container and refrigerate.

Tomato Dressing

This a delicious dressing with a balance of sweetness and acidity – it will work very nicely with fish or salad.

150 ml olive oil
1 punnet of cherry tomatoes
⅓ bunch of basil
40 ml red wine vinegar
¼ red onion, finely chopped
sea salt and freshly ground black pepper, to taste

1   Place a small saucepan over medium heat and add the olive oil. Add the tomatoes and simmer for 6–8 minutes. Remove from the heat and allow to cool.

2   Place the tomatoes in a blender or food processor with the remaining ingredients and lightly blitz for 10–20 seconds, or until smooth.

3   Season again with salt and pepper if needed, and serve.

makes
1
cup

Chimichurri

This is one of my all-time favourite dressings; it goes well with most dishes. If you like it as much as me, I recommend making a large batch and storing it in the fridge.

½ bunch of coriander
½ bunch of parsley
3–5 mint leaves
1 green chilli
5 tablespoons olive oil
2 tablespoons red wine vinegar
sea salt and freshly ground black pepper,
   to taste

1   Throw all the ingredients in a blender or food processor and blitz for 30 seconds, or until fully combined.

2   Transfer to an airtight container and store in the fridge.

makes
3
cups

Keto Satay Sauce

Once you make this you'll be making it frequently, for one good reason – it's YUM!

2 cups raw macadamias
½ cup coconut milk
1 teaspoon fish sauce
1 long red chilli, deseeded and chopped
2 teaspoons lime juice
1 teaspoon honey
sea salt and freshly ground black pepper,
   to taste

1   Throw all the ingredients in a blender or food processor and blitz for 20–30 seconds, or until smooth.

2   Season again with salt and pepper if needed, and serve.

makes 1/2 cup

Tahini Dressing

This dressing goes well with fish, veggies or salad and is ridiculously simple to make.

2 tablespoons tahini
½ garlic clove, minced
juice of 1 lemon
½ tsp cumin
⅓ cup water
sea salt and freshly ground black pepper, to taste

1   In a mixing bowl, combine the tahini and minced garlic. Add the lemon juice and cumin, and stir.

2   Slowly stir in the water until desired consistency is reached. Season to taste with salt and pepper.

makes 500 ml

Green Tahini

Tahini is a great ingredient to have in the cupboard. It's perfect for adding to smoothies or ice-creams but similarly can be a dressing or a dip very easily.

225 ml tahini
125 ml water
1 tablespoon minced garlic
juice of 2 lemons
handful of baby spinach leaves
½ bunch of parsley
½ bunch of coriander
100 ml olive oil
sea salt and freshly ground black pepper, to taste

1   Throw all the ingredients in a blender or food processor and blitz for 20–30 seconds, or until fully combined.

2   Season again with salt and pepper if needed, then transfer to an airtight container and store in the fridge.

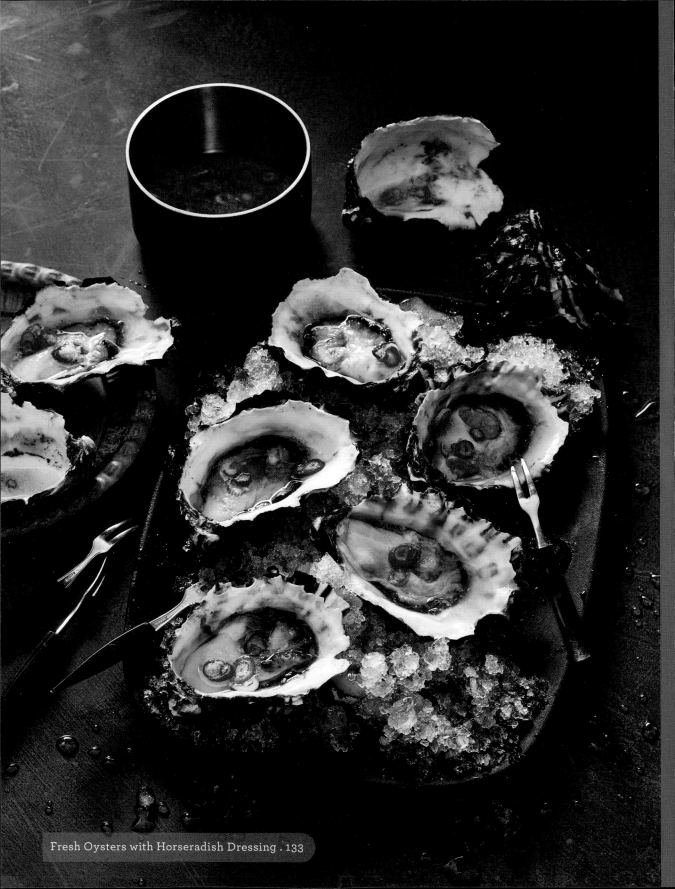

Fresh Oysters with Horseradish Dressing . 133

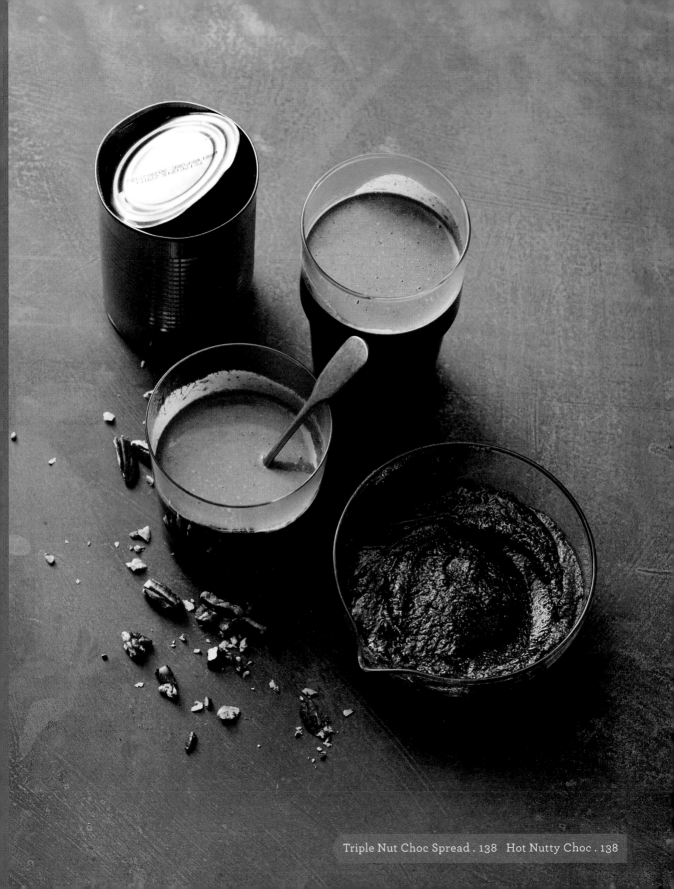

Triple Nut Choc Spread . 138   Hot Nutty Choc . 138

makes
2

Super Veg Smoothie

This smoothie is a real powerhouse for health, with some potent and nutrient-dense ingredients. This recipe works well for an up-and-go, if you're pushed for time in the mornings, and it's also fab for kids.

1 red capsicum, deseeded
1 large tomato
2 cm knob of ginger
2 cm knob of turmeric
3 cups chopped kale leaves
1 cup baby spinach leaves
1 small baby beetroot, trimmed
1 tablespoon MCT oil
300 ml coconut milk
100 ml water

1   Throw all the ingredients in a blender and blitz for 20 seconds, or until fully combined.

2   Pour into glasses and serve.

serves
1–2

Gut-healing Smoothie

Don't be alarmed at seeing broth in my smoothie recipe, it's included for its therapeutic properties.

250 ml coconut milk
50 ml chicken broth or stock
½ ripe avocado, flesh scooped out
   (can be frozen)
50 ml coconut kefir
30 g vanilla protein powder
1 tablespoon MCT oil
50 g raw macadamias
handful of ice

1   Throw all the ingredients in a blender and blitz for 20–30 seconds, or until fully combined.

2   Pour into a glass or glasses, and serve.

theketodietcookbook

serves
2

Protein Smoothie

Collagen is a potent ingredient to help with soft tissue repair, as well as being beneficial for gut health. Collagen can be added to a smoothie without greatly affecting its overall flavour.

400 ml coconut milk
1 cup frozen blueberries
1 cup frozen or fresh baby spinach leaves
2 egg yolks
1 tablespoon nut butter of your choice
2 tablespoons collagen powder
1 teaspoon honey (optional)
handful of ice

1   Throw all the ingredients in a blender and blitz for 20 seconds, or until fully combined.

2   Pour into glasses and serve.

serves
1

Bulletproof Broth

Most commercial bone broths are low in fat (it's deliberately removed), so amplify your quick and easy broth recipe by adding some veggies and fat.

300 ml chicken broth
1 teaspoon MCT oil
1 teaspoon ghee
1 carrot, diced
1 cup chopped spinach
sea salt and freshly ground black pepper, to taste

1   Place the broth in a small saucepan and bring to the boil. Once boiling, remove from the heat and transfer to a blender.

2   Add the remaining ingredients and blitz for 20 seconds (ensure the lid is on securely).

3   Season again with salt and pepper if needed, and serve.

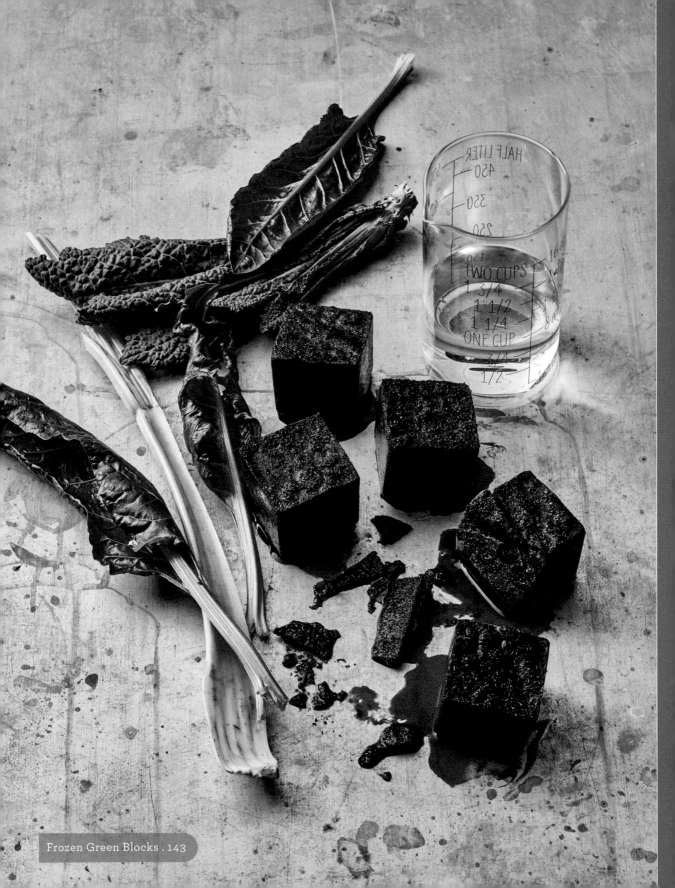

serves
2

Turmeric Spiced Latte

300 ml coconut milk
1 cinnamon stick
½ teaspoon turmeric
½ teaspoon allspice
½ teaspoon honey

1   Combine all the ingredients in a small saucepan over low heat. Lightly simmer for 7–8 minutes, stirring occasionally.

2   Remove the cinnamon stick, pour into mugs and serve.

serves
1

Bulletproof Matcha Green Tea

Matcha is an incredibly potent antioxidant and anti-ageing tea leaf. This version of the bulletproof drink has the caffeine equivalent of half a standard coffee.

2 matcha green tea bags
1 tablespoon butter
1–2 teaspoons MCT oil

1   Brew your green tea as per usual, then transfer to a blender and add the butter and MCT oil. Blitz for 20 seconds (ensure the lid is on securely).

2   Pour into a mug or glass, and serve.

makes
6
ice-cubes

Frozen Green Blocks

A large part of adhering to a healthy lifestyle is being prepared. With these blocks in your freezer you'll be the envy of any boy or girl scout. Use them to add to smoothies.

1 bunch of English spinach
6 kale leaves, trimmed
1 celery stalk
½ cup water

1   Throw all the ingredients in a blender and blitz for 20–30 seconds, or until fully combined.

2   Pour into large ice-cube trays and pop into the freezer for a minimum of 2 hours.

3   Add a green block to your smoothie.

Raspberry and Chocolate Ice-cream . 147   Blueberry and Chocolate Ice-cream . 147

Raspberry and Chocolate Ice-cream

If you want to add some texture to the ice-cream you can sprinkle a little toasted granola on top – see recipe on page 9.

4 whole eggs
4 egg yolks
2 teaspoons vanilla extract
1 teaspoon apple cider vinegar or lime juice
3 tablespoons coconut oil
3 tablespoons MCT oil
100 g softened butter
¾ cup frozen raspberries
½ cup cacao powder
1 teaspoon honey
fresh berries, to serve

1   Throw all the ingredients except the fresh berries in a blender and blitz for 10–20 seconds, or until the mixture is lump-free.

2   Transfer to a freezer-safe container, cover and place in the freezer.

3   Remove from the freezer 5–10 minutes before serving. Top with fresh berries.

Blueberry and Chocolate Ice-cream

This recipe rocks my world. I stand by every ingredient and can honestly say it's good for you!

4 whole eggs
4 egg yolks
2 teaspoons vanilla extract
1 teaspoon apple cider vinegar or lime juice
3 tablespoons coconut oil
3 tablespoons MCT oil
100 g softened butter
¾ cup frozen blueberries
½ cup cacao powder
1 teaspoon honey
fresh berries, to serve

1   Throw all the ingredients except the fresh berries in a blender and blitz for 10–20 seconds, or until the mixture is lump-free.

2   Transfer to a freezer-safe container, cover and place in the freezer.

3   Remove from the freezer 5–10 minutes before serving. Top with fresh berries.

Chocolate Mousse Torte with Mixed Berries

Healthy treats can be a grey area for health, but this is good recipe to roll out for someone's birthday. But treats should always be just that … a treat.

2 cups almond meal
½ cup cacao powder, plus ⅓ cup extra
   for the mousse
½ cup melted coconut oil
2 ripe avocados, flesh scooped out
½ cup desiccated coconut
⅓ cup honey
1 teaspoon vanilla extract
¾ cup coconut cream
100 g blueberries
50 g raspberries

1   In a large mixing bowl, combine the almond meal, ½ cup cacao powder and coconut oil.

2   Using a 20 cm wide × 3 cm deep fluted tin with a removable base, press the mixture into the base and sides. Chill in the fridge for a minimum of 1 hour.

3   Place the avocado, desiccated coconut, honey, vanilla, coconut cream and ⅓ cup cacao powder in a blender and blitz until smooth.

4   Fill the tart base with the mousse and return to the fridge for a further 30 minutes.

5   Top with the berries before serving.

Mixed Berries with Lemon Coconut Cream

Sometimes the desire to have something sweet is hard to ignore. Rather than reaching out for something unhealthy, try this recipe!

1 × 400 ml can coconut cream, chilled
juice of ½ lemon
grated zest of 1 lemon
½ cup blueberries
¼ cup raspberries
¼ cup blackberries

1   Refrigerate the coconut cream can for a minimum of 1 hour.

2   Take the can out of the fridge, open and remove the watery component.

3   Place the coconut cream (solids) in a mixing bowl. Add the lemon juice and zest and whisk to combine.

4   Place the mixed berries in serving bowls and top each bowl with 1 tablespoon of the lemon coconut cream.

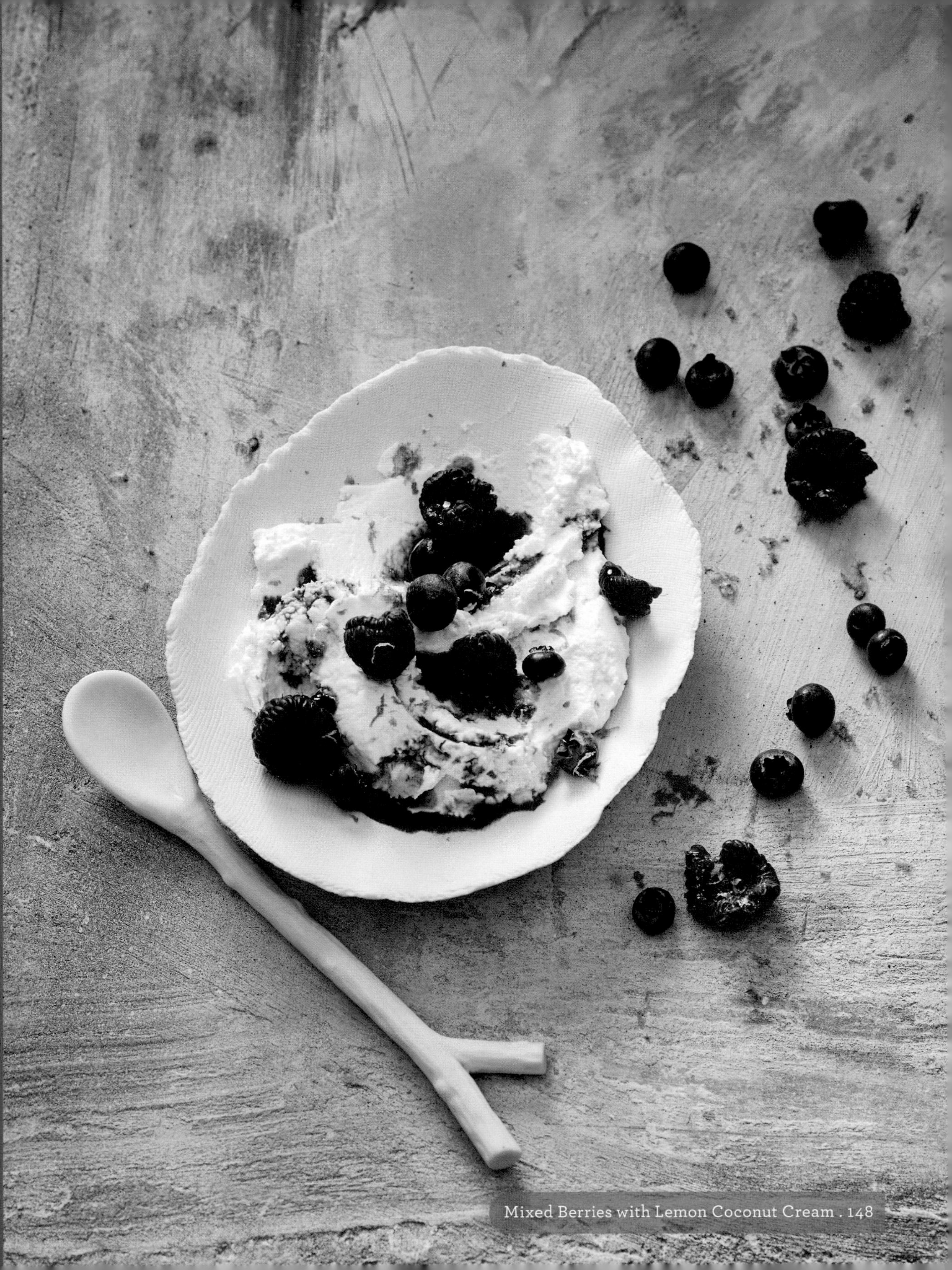

Mixed Berries with Lemon Coconut Cream . 148

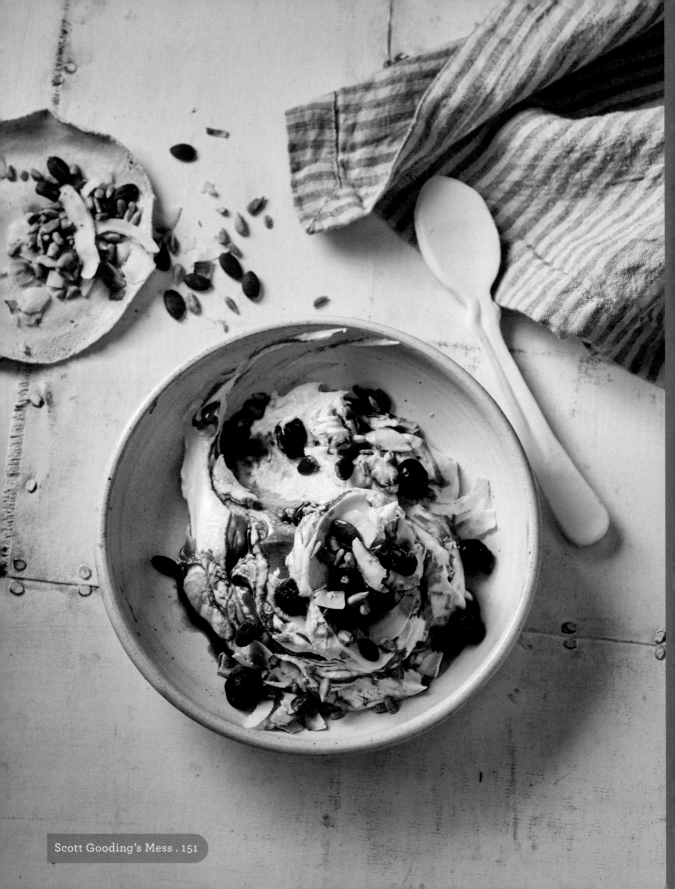

serves
1

Scott Gooding's Mess

We eat with our eyes, I know, and presentation is everything, BUT throw that out the window for now. This is my version of a little treat after dinner … it is not that easy on the eye, but it hits the spot taste-wise!

¼ cup frozen blueberries
1 tablespoon, peanut butter or nut butter
  of your choice
1 tablespoon shredded coconut
1–2 tablespoons coconut cream
1 tablespoon pepitas
1 tablespoon sunflower seeds
1 tablespoon MCT oil (optional)

1   Combine all the ingredients in a bowl
    and serve.

RECIPE INDEX